W9-BSM-951

"Jon Barron is probably the greatest mind in alternative health today."

Roy Brabham, M.D., Baton Rouge, LA

"I wouldn't be alive today without *Lessons from the Miracle Doctors* and the Baseline of Health."

Howard Ritter, Pryor, OK

"This is nothing short of a miracle. I have my life back. If you or someone you know or love needs help, I urge you to take a serious look at this program."

Sue Ellen Dickinson, Ft. Walton Beach, FL

"Thanks to Jon Barron's book, *Lessons from the Miracle Doctors,* I have my life back."

Nina Embrey, Diamond, MO

"I have always been a strong advocate and firm believer in health promotion and disease prevention, and I believe Jon Barron's program will achieve this goal. I am convinced that *Lessons from the Miracle Doctors* has life-changing potential, and I am 100% committed to it and will do everything in my power to share this information with others."

Badi Jeffers M.D., Orange County, CA

"Many people who have subscribed to his newsletters over the years already know that Jon is probably the best writer on alternative health in the world today. *Lessons from the Miracle Doctors* can only serve to cement that reputation even further."

Ron Manwarren, President, Royal Botanicals, Los Angeles, CA

Lessons from the Miracle Doctors

by Jon Barron

Healing America, Inc.

Medicine is, and always should be, considered a vast field of service, constantly pioneering to improve the well-being of us all. From the beginning of my education in health and nutrition, I have known many medical doctors whose efforts and service to humanity could be described as nothing less than heroic.

It is with these doctors (and that perspective) in mind that I offer this book to any and all who read it. This book is dedicated to all those who have fought ignorance and prejudice, to all those who have paid the price, and to keeping this information alive and available for the rest of us. Among a whole host of others, these include Dr. John Christopher, Sandra Michael, Dr. Richard Schultz, Dr. Julian Whitaker, Dr. David Williams, Dr. Jonathan Wright, and my wife, Kristen.

Copyright © 1999, Jon Barron.

All rights reserved. No part of this book may be reproduced, stored in a retrieval system, or transmitted by any means, electronic, mechanical, photocopying, recording, or otherwise, without written permission from the author. Although every precaution has been taken in the preparation of this book, the publisher and author assume no responsibility for errors or omissions. Neither is any liability assumed for damages resulting from the use of the information contained herein.

First Printing May, 1999

Second Printing July, 1999

Third Printing August, 1999

Fourth Printing May, 2000

Fifth Printing April, 2001

Sixth Printing April, 2002

Seventh Printing August 2002

ISBN 0-9719198-0-1

Distributed by Healing America, Inc.

CONTENTS

Foreword

The variety of pain and suffering is as plentiful and as diverse as humankind. Sickness, disease, and injury abound, and the world cries for help. Throughout the ages, we have found comfort in our healers, our doctors and nurses—individuals who give their very lives to solace our grief and bind up our hurt. They have become bigger than life, and in the truest sense, they are heroes.

In America, we have grown up trusting our family doctor. There is peace of mind in knowing that someone cares, that someone knows your child by name and is moved by compassion when you, or someone you love, is hurting.

In my life and travels around this globe, I have met many great healers. I have seen them at their best and marveled at their skill and courage. In emergency rooms and intensive care units, in private clinics and at disaster sites, in burn units and trauma centers, they work tirelessly with heart and hand. They save lives and mend bodies, unite loved ones and offer hope. Our world is better because of them.

Understand, when you need a doctor, only a doctor will do. If you are severely injured in an automobile accident, you want a skilled surgeon—not even the best herbalist in the world will do.

Modern medical science has made incredible advances and contributions which have alleviated pain and suffering. Surgical technique (the cutting apart and repairing of the human body) has made remarkable progress. Identification of germs that cause disease and improved sanitation, which aids in preventing that disease, have also seen vast achievements. Burn treatment, trauma, and emergency room care are nothing less than miraculous. When it comes to these areas of medical care, the value they bring to us is impossible to measure.

But as you read the pages of this book and note my candid observations, you will see that there is another side to this story. There is great failure in health care today—and, as a result of that failure, great pain and unnecessary suffering. And it is important that as you discover how badly the modern medical paradigm is failing that you take great care not to assign blame wrongly. Yes, there are doctors whose practices we all abhor, and we wish they could never practice medicine again; this book is not for them, and it is not about them. Neither is my commentary directed at the thousands of faithful health care workers who go about their daily jobs. Specifically, I am driven to confront the very foundation of the modern medical paradigm, a philosophy that costs trillions, promises hope, but delivers misery. No one, including many inside the influential medical community, can help but acknowledge these great failings. The bottom line is that if modern medicine had been effective in addressing the major and most threatening scourges of our time (heart disease, cancer, diabetes, osteoporosis, Alzheimer's, etc.), this book would have no purpose. But sadly, for all our education and massive expenditures, modern medicine has failed miserably. You may wonder why.

Modern medicine likes to trace its roots to Hippocrates, the patron saint of today's doctors. In truth, its roots rest more comfortably in the Newtonian views of the 17th century when philosophers and scientists defined the universe as a great machine. Physicians of that era were not immune to this influence and likewise began to define the human body as a machine. According to this "new" paradigm, the body could be analyzed, catalogued, adjusted, and repaired as required—just like any other machine.

This viewpoint became firmly established during the 19th century when the "body as machine" concept was taken to its ultimate, absurd extreme. The human body was no longer viewed as a holistic entity, but rather as a grouping of separate parts and pieces. Disease was no longer viewed as a body state, but as a set of symptoms. Ultimately, and so it is today, the province of medicine has become the observation and classification (or at least the management) of those symptoms. In this paradigm, disease or illness or injury manifests itself as symptoms entirely separate from the body as a whole (a decidedly nonholistic paradigm). The body is irrelevant. If the symptom can be eliminated (i.e., the pain and suffering), the problem must of necessity be gone as well.[1]

As it turns out, this paradigm works very well in surgical repair. If you break an arm, the doctor works with that part of the machine and repairs your arm. If you are wounded by a bullet, the doctor removes the bullet and repairs all of the separate parts of your body damaged by the bullet—again, problem solved!

Unfortunately, the paradigm fails when it comes to the major diseases of our time—cancer, heart disease, diabetes, Alzheimer's, etc. Consider:

- You have clogged arteries. This eventually causes your blood pressure to rise, so your doctor prescribes blood pressure medication to eliminate the symptom of high blood pressure—not the problem, clogged arteries. To reduce blood pressure, doctors have essentially four classes of medication in their arsenal.

1. **Diuretics,** which reduce pressure by making you pee out water from your body. Reduce the volume of fluid in your blood, and you reduce the pressure. Unfortunately, side effects can include dizziness, weakness, an increased risk of strokes, and impotence. (Not to worry, there are medications to alleviate the side effects.)

---

[1]And there are some who would argue that today's medicine has even gone beyond treating the body as a machine—that doctors, today, have taken things to whole new levels of absurdity; they treat the body as a mere set of "numbers." Consider this: When you go to your doctor now, he or she orders up a series of very expensive tests (bloodwork, PSA, EEG, etc.), each of which produces a set of numbers. Then, based on those numbers, your doctor prescribes a series of drugs to move those numbers up or down. In this model, even symptoms don't matter—only the numbers.

2. **Calcium channel blockers,** which work to relax and widen the arteries—thus reducing blood pressure. Then again, a major side effect of channel blockers is a 60% increased risk of heart attack.
3. **Beta blockers,** which work by weakening the heart so it won't pump as strongly, thereby reducing blood pressure. One of the major problems with beta blockers, though, is the increased risk of congestive heart failure. Now catch this. Despite the increased risk of congestive heart failure, an article in the *New England Journal of Medicine* (August 20, 1998), recommended putting "every single" heart attack survivor on beta blockers.
4. **ACE inhibitors** (the new drugs of choice), which like the calcium channel blockers, also work to relax and widen the arteries. Unfortunately, ACE inhibitors can produce severe allergic reactions, can be deadly to fetuses and children who are breastfeeding, and can cause severe kidney damage.

But remember, these drugs only treat the symptom, not the cause—clogged arteries. So eventually, as your arteries continue to clog to the point where even the medication no longer helps, you start getting the inevitable chest pains and shortness of breath. At that point, your doctor is then forced to chase the next set of symptoms and perform a coronary bypass or angioplasty to relieve the symptoms.

And like the drugs before it, surgery merely addresses the symptoms, not the problem. Think about this for a moment: If all your doctor did was bypass or clear the arteries supplying blood to your heart, doesn't that mean that all of the other arteries in your body are still clogged—including the arteries that supply blood to your brain? The answer, of course, is yes. And, in fact, your odds of having a stroke after heart surgery are dramatically increased.

Not to worry. Your doctor has another drug to deal with this problem: Coumadin® (medicinal rat poison), which inhibits clotting and thins your blood so that it flows more easily through the narrowed arteries. But Coumadin has its own set of problems, and, of course, you are still on all of the previous blood-pressure drugs and symptom relieving drugs that your doctor previously prescribed.

The bottom line is that the average person 65 years or older in the United States takes an average of 15+ medications a day (prescription and over-the-counter combined), each and every day of their lives. And only the first 1 or 2 drugs are actually prescribed to deal with the original medical problem. The other 13+ drugs are all required to deal with the negative side effects of the original 2, plus the interactions of all the other drugs they are taking. And the really sad fact is that in over 95% of all cases, the original problem could have been resolved naturally—with no side effects.

Do you understand the implications of that statement?

Disease can be averted, treated, and in many, many cases even reversed—naturally, with no side effects!

I have been fortunate to travel the world, to meet and spend time with dedicated men and women (some from within the medical community, and some from the world of holistic medicine) whose work in the field of healing has distinguished them as miracle doctors. Not once or twice, but every day, over and over, they do what modern medicine says is impossible. They cure the incurable.

I found these remarkable people to be open and willing to share their ideas and methods, and they found me hungry to learn. I have seen firsthand the evidence of their work. In addition to watching and listening, I have read and researched, catalogued and compared, and finally assembled here in these pages principles that can make you well…and keep you well.

These are not untried theories. I have not sought after fads or latest trends. Many of the truths included here are centuries old. All are proven. Good health is not the result of any single action. There are no"magic bullets" when it comes to achieving good health. Good health is the result of making right decisions day after beautiful day.

In the pages that follow, I have tried to show you the barriers to obtaining good health, and I have presented practical, proven step-by-step methods for breaking down those barriers and seizing (for yourself and your family) health, energy, and mental and spiritual well-being. A lot of what you will learn here will fly in the face of so-called "conventional wisdom." But understand, just because something is commonly accepted does not necessarily make it true. Our modern society has invested countless trillions of dollars into the ideas, equipment, research, facilities, and promises of our present health care system, and it is almost unbearable to consider that much of it is a waste. It will take great courage to accept responsibility for your own health, but I believe you, and millions like you, can, and will, do just that.

It has often been said that this is the only body you'll ever get, and it must last a lifetime. The only question is how long and healthy that life will be. The simple fact is that you absolutely can live well into your 70s, 80s, and beyond, in great health and with great vitality—but you need to make the right decisions now for that to happen. If you want to live a full and satisfying life, then you must take back control of your own health—today.

Jon Barron

CHAPTER 1

THERE HAS TO BE AN ALTERNATIVE

Thirty years ago, diseases such as colon cancer, prostate cancer, and diverticular disease were virtually unknown. Today, they are almost a certainty if you live long enough.[1] Consider:

What We Pay for Health Care

- Never in the history of the world has any other country come close to having as many doctors as we do in the United States: approximately 700,000 according to the US Census.
- And never in the entire history of the world has any other country come close to spending as much as we do on health care: a conservative one trillion dollars a year. That means that what we spend on health care is more than the entire Gross National Product of all but six countries in the world today.[2]

What Value Have We Received?

- We lead the developed world in deaths from
  - Heart disease
  - Prostate cancer
  - Breast cancer
  - Colorectal cancer
  - Diabetes
- The American Cancer Society now says that one in every 2.5 individuals will develop some form of invasive cancer during their lifetime—and half of them will die from it.
- Cancer is the leading cause of death by disease in children under the age of 10.

---

[1]Sources for statistics are endless, and, depending on what source is used, actual numbers may vary. But regardless of how the numbers may vary, two things remain constant: the steadily increasing trend of major diseases (such as heart disease, cancer, diabetes, and infectious diseases) and the exponentially rising costs associated with those diseases.

[2]Figures for the amount spent on health care in the United States range from $1–$1.4 trillion per year. But even at the lower $1-trillion figure, that's still more than **the total GNP** of 124 out of the world's 130 countries.

- And even though we spend 100 billion dollars a year on cancer treatment and research, the overall survival rate for cancer patients is **no better** than it was 50 or 100 years ago.

And It's Getting Worse

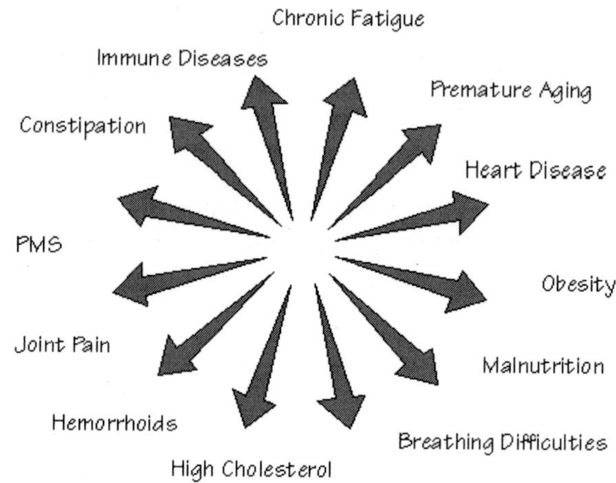

- The incidence of diabetes in the United States has **doubled** in just the **last 5 years!**
- Fifty years ago, diverticular disease (herniations of the colon) was virtually unknown (afflicting less than 10% of the American population). Today, according to the Merck Manual, 100% of all Americans will have many—if they live long enough.
- Thirty years ago, colorectal cancer was virtually unknown. Today, it is the single most prevalent cancer among men and women combined.
- The number of Americans who suffer from Asthma, according to the Centers for Disease Control, has risen by an astounding 75% in just the last 20 years.
- Breast cancer rates are up 30% in just the last 15 years.
- And on . . . and on . . . and on
- And now it's official: In the February 9, 1994 issue of the *Journal of the American Medical Association,* the "War on Cancer" was declared a failure. "In all age groups, cancer incidence is increasing . . . Few new, effective treatments have been devised for the most common cancers."

And the Most Shocking Fact of All

The April 15, 1998 *Journal of the American Medical Association* reported that there are more than 2,000,000 drug "reactions" annually in the United States, and that more than 100,000 of those reactions are fatal. This makes prescription drugs the fourth leading cause of death in America. But the reality is actually far worse.

- These numbers **only** count drugs that are prescribed correctly and at the right dose.
- **Not included** are patients who are given the wrong drugs, or who are given those drugs at the wrong dosage or in the wrong combination.
- And these numbers do not include the patients who have fatal reactions to the drugs, but whose deaths are mistakenly attributed to other causes.
- Nor do these numbers include the patients whose cause of death is deliberately obscured to protect the physicians and hospitals involved.
  - Add in these numbers, and you find that deaths from adverse reactions to drugs may number as high as 700,000 a year. (Actually, the FDA estimates that only 1% of all adverse reactions are reported[1]—which, if true, would make 700,000 a very conservative estimate.) And finally, combine that 700,000 with the number of people who die from misdiagnosis, inappropriate treatment, secondary infections received in hospitals, or just plain physician error,[2] and the startling fact you're left with is that **the modern medical paradigm, despite all its accomplishments, is arguably the single leading cause of death in the United States.**

Understand, this is **not** an attack on medical doctors—the vast majority of whom are extremely competent, highly dedicated, and (as I mentioned earlier) often even heroic. Nevertheless, it is important to realize that when it comes to the major diseases of our time, the modern medical paradigm of searching for "magic bullets" and managing symptoms with drugs has failed miserably.

There Has to Be an Alternative!

There is a network of elite herbalists, holistic healers, and renegade medical doctors throughout the world, performing miracles on a daily basis. The network is not only elite, it is also extremely difficult to penetrate because it is technically illegal to diagnose or treat people for major diseases unless you use the FDA approved modalities such as Cutting, Burning, and Poisoning (surgery, radiation, and chemo). **Thousands of people throughout the world have come to these "miracle doctors" terminally ill, and thousands have left healthy. And now the secrets of these "Miracle Doctors" are revealed in this book.**

[1]A study by a group of French doctors actually makes that 1% estimate seem wildly optimistic. The study found that only about **1 out of every 24,000** adverse reactions is actually reported by doctors to the appropriate monitoring agency.

[2]Just one example of how high these numbers actually are: On the ABC News *Nightline* program, the Harvard School of Public Health stated that approximately 1.3 million people a year suffer some kind of injury because of hospital treatment, and 180,000 of those people die.

In the following pages, I will share with you those things that I have learned in my 30+ years of working with, studying with, and sharing with these remarkable healers. By the time you have finished, you will have learned everything you need to know (in precise detail) to optimize your own health (and the health of those you know and love) and to live a long and happy life.

1. In the next chapter, I will outline the principles of **The Baseline of Health.** If you read no other chapter in this book, the heart of everything I have to say is located here.
2. The rest of the chapters in the book address all of the different body systems you need to concern yourself with in order to optimize your health—and give you step-by-step pointers on how to accomplish just that.
3. In conclusion, I will provide you with very specific product and usage recommendations.

   Note: Keep in mind that good health really comes down to "playing the odds."

- For example, if you smoke cigarettes, there's no guarantee that you're going to get sick and die. (We've all heard stories of the man who smoked and drank like a fiend for 80 years, only to be shot to death by a jealous husband when the smoker was discovered in bed with the other man's 20-year-old wife.) On the other hand, there's no question that your "odds" of having emphysema or lung cancer or of having parts of your mouth, lips, and tongue surgically removed increase dramatically if you smoke. It's all a question of "odds."
- Well, in the same way, if you follow the program laid down in this book, your "odds" of having good health and long life are significantly increased—not guaranteed, but significantly increased. Oh yes, and you're going to feel a whole lot better, have more energy, vitality, sexuality, youthfulness, and radiance in the process.

Good Health and Long Life

CHAPTER 2

THE BASELINE OF HEALTH

Magical Herbs

Over the years, I've lectured to thousands of people, and thousands more have read my newsletters; and, even though my message is always based on the same principle espoused by all of the miracle doctors (that the body is a holistic system and needs to be treated as such), after every lecture, after every newsletter is mailed, I nevertheless receive dozens and dozens of requests from people desperately looking for that "magic herb" (or supplement) to "cure" themselves or their loved ones of some dreaded disease. The problem is that health doesn't work like that. First, the concept of the magic herb or supplement is a myth (more on this in a moment), and second, the legal system takes a dim view of espousing specific "cures" that do not fall within the mainstream of modern medicine.

Now for the good news! It doesn't matter. Everything you need to know is totally laid out in the Baseline of Health Program.

Mystical Body

Getting rid of disease is not the big problem (doctors do it all the time). The problem is making sure the disease doesn't return. (Something doctors don't do quite as well.) And this is where The Baseline of Health Program comes in. This program is the synthesis of all the best that is taught by today's miracle doctors. The program is designed to empower your own body to throw off illness and keep the illness from returning. Variations of this program have proven so effective that hundreds of thousands of people have experienced remarkable healings by using it.

THE BASELINE OF HEALTH

Before we can understand the program that is based on it, we first have to understand what the Baseline of Health actually is. For purposes of our discussion, we will use a simple X-Y chart to represent the state of our health. The Y axis represents the level of our health. And on the X axis, we have all the systems and organs that affect our health. These actually number in the hundreds (if not thousands), but to keep things simple on our chart, we'll just list three: the Immune System, the Circulatory System, and Control of Mutated Cells.

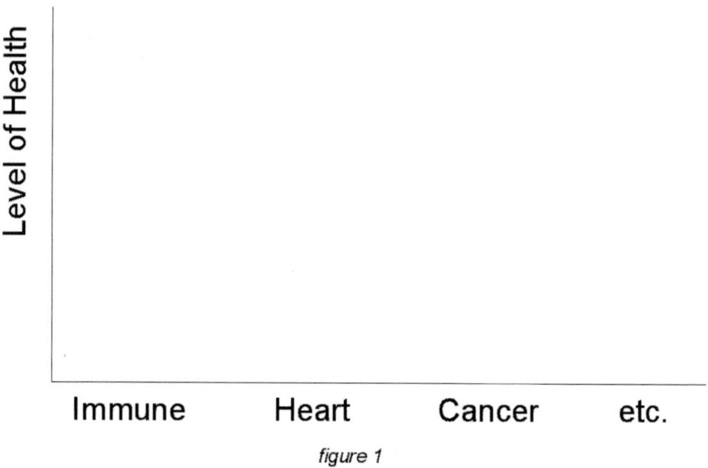

figure 1

For all these systems and organs there are only three lines that we are concerned with:

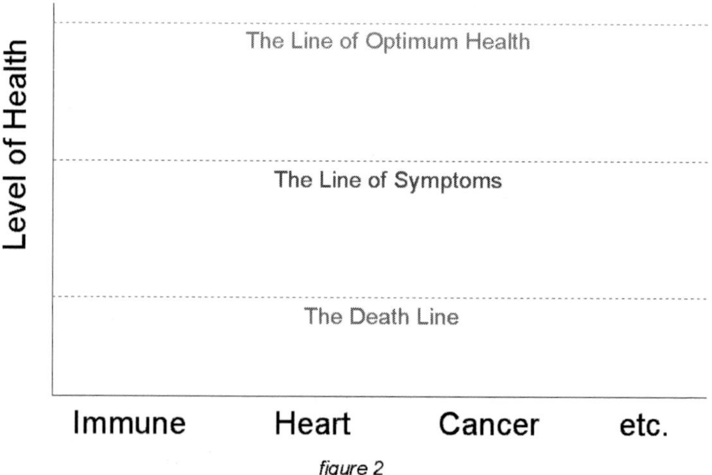

figure 2

- **The Line of Optimum Health.** In a perfect world, our Personal Health Line would match the Line of Optimum Health. In reality, that's not achievable. So what we try to do is keep everything as close to Optimum Health as possible.
- **The Line of Symptoms.** As long as all our organs and systems function above this line, we have no problems. But the moment any part of our Personal Health Line dips below the Line of Symptoms, problems begin to manifest. Sometimes, the problems are so slight we don't notice them at first—such as the early warning signals of heart disease and cancer. But at a certain point, if the symptoms persist long enough, and if our Personal Health Line dips below the Line of Symptoms far enough, we take notice.
- **The Death Line.** If any part of our Personal Health Line touches the Death Line, we die.

Now let's take a look at this concept in action. As an example, we'll track the case history of Jim, an average 40-year-old American. Below is Jim's Personal Health Line at birth.

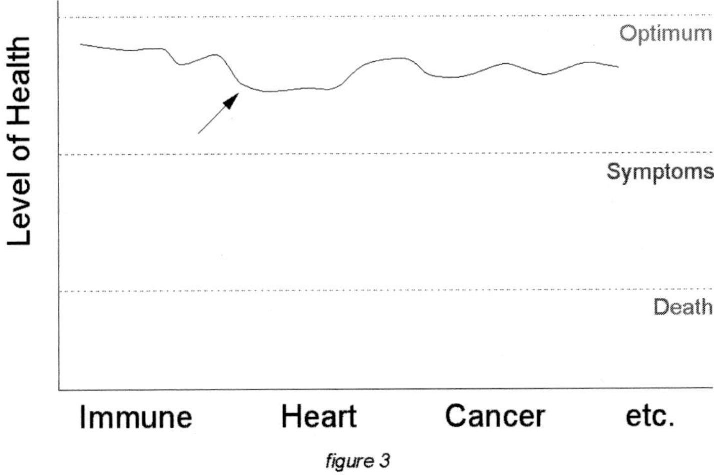

figure 3

As we can see from Jim's line above, he was born with a slight weakness (either genetic or as a result of his parents' lifestyle and environment) in his heart and circulatory system. Note also, that at birth, Jim is in relatively good health and is symptom free (as no point of his Personal Health Line dips below the Line of Symptoms).

Over the 40 years of his life, however, Jim has contributed to that weakness in his heart and circulatory system because of a diet high in hydrogenated oils and refined carbohydrates, a folic acid deficiency, a low pH, and **heavy free radical damage**—to the point where his Personal Health Line has dipped below the Line of Symptoms.

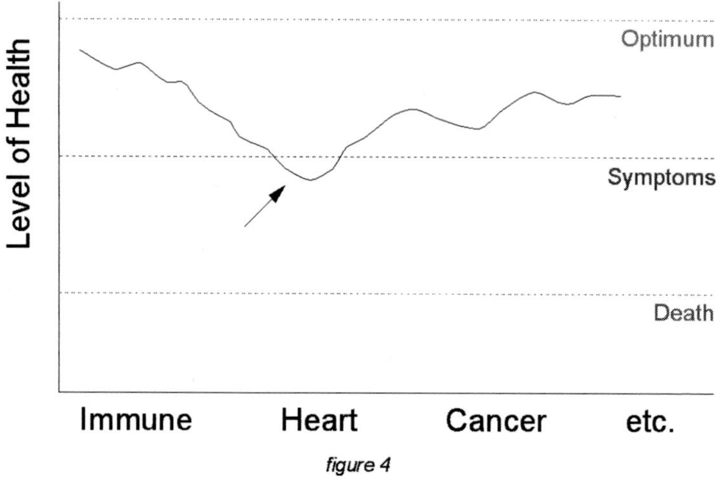

figure 4

A friend of Jim's suggests he try an antioxidant supplement. Since the antioxidant addresses one of Jim's problems (free radical damage), Jim's Personal Health Line once again rises above the Line of Symptoms (even if just by a little bit) and all of Jim's symptoms disappear.

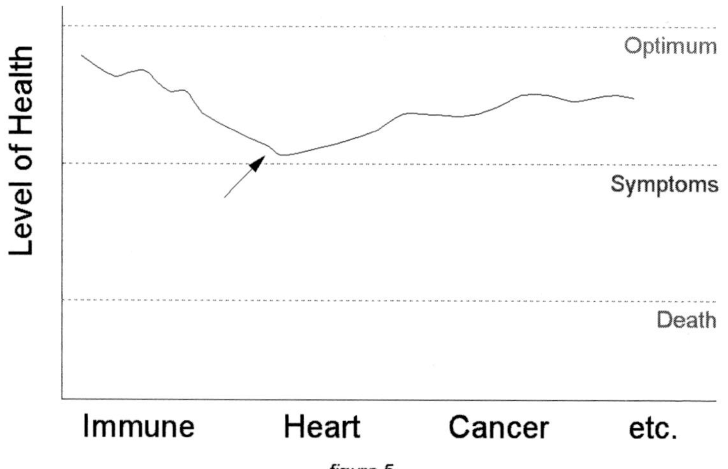

figure 5

"It's a miracle! All of my symptoms are gone. I'm cured. If you have any heart problems, or any health problems at all, you must try this supplement." Jim is so excited, he decides to promote the antioxidant company and proceeds to sell his miracle cure to everyone he meets.

One day, he talks to Mary, who also has heart problems. Like Jim, Mary too was born with a predilection to heart problems; and like Jim she has managed to exacerbate that problem through folic acid deficiency, low pH, and a **high stress work environment.**

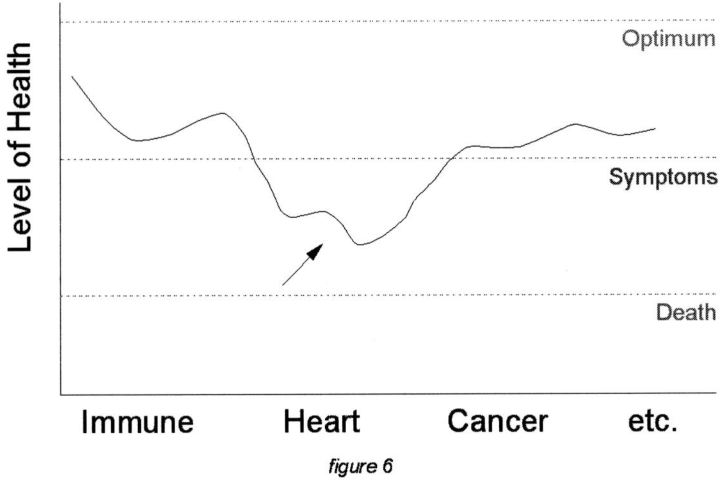

figure 6

Jim convinces Mary to buy a supply of his "miracle" antioxidant; and, as recommended by Jim, Mary starts gulping down handfuls of her daily dose. But remember, unlike Jim, Mary has very little free radical damage. (Let's say she loves Italian food with real olive oil and red wine—two foods that, over the years, have mitigated any free radical damage she might have been exposed to.) The net result is that Mary notices no change in her condition (see figure 7).

Mary now proceeds to tell Jim that he's crazy. Whatever benefit he got from the antioxidant is purely a placebo effect. It's a waste of money. Of course, later on, when Mary enters a stress management program, or has heart bypass surgery, she now tells everyone she knows that she's found the *real* cure for heart disease and recommends to all her friends that they do the same. (It's worth noting that the antioxidant did, in fact, significantly improve the overall level of her Personal Health Line, but since Mary didn't feel any difference, she incorrectly assumed that she had received no benefit.)

The bottom line is that the same supplement, used by two different people

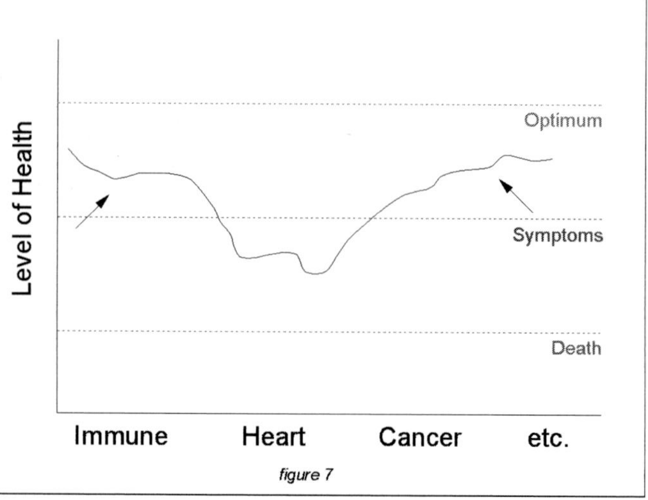

figure 7

for the same condition, produced two entirely different results. What does that mean? It means that gulping down "miracle herbs" and "miracle supplements" to treat disease is like trying to hit a clay pigeon in the sky, with a 22-caliber rifle . . . while blindfolded. The odds are very much against you.

The secret to health, the secret to all of the success that the great alternative healers share, is that they look to raise every inch of a person's Personal Health Line. If you do that, if you raise the entire line, the odds are in your favor. In fact, it's almost impossible to miss. Specifically, the body systems and topics that we're going to address throughout the rest of this book are:

1. **Intestinal cleansing, detoxification, and rebuilding.** Cleaning out the elimination channels is fundamental to any health building program.

2. **Probiotics.** As a result of chlorinated/fluorinated/treated water and antibiotics and pesticides in our food, we have virtually eliminated an essential component of health and well-being. There can be no true health or relief from disease until we rebuild it.

3. **Enzymes.** Modern man is the only animal that eats a diet almost entirely devoid of live enzymes. As a result, virtually every American has an enlarged pancreas by the time he/she is 40 and a significantly diminished life expectancy.

4. **Diet.** Every cell, every system, every organ in our bodies is produced from the food we eat. Sorry, but you can't make a healthy body from a diet predominantly comprised of potato chips and diet soda.

5. **Vitamins, Minerals, and Phytochemicals.** Supplementation of some kind

is mandatory. But with so many products and companies pitching the next wonder supplement, how can you tell which is best?

6. **Herbs.** The great herbalists don't just cure colds; they cure cancer!

7. **Free Radicals and Antioxidants.** Scientists now know that free radicals play a major role in the aging process as well as in the onset of cancer, heart disease, stroke, arthritis, and possibly allergies and a host of other ailments. But which antioxidants work best for you?

8. **Hormonal Balance.** Each and every day we are exposed to thousands and thousands and thousands of chemicals that work to destroy the hormonal balance of our bodies—with disastrous effects. Correcting these imbalances can save our health—and our sanity!!

9. **Water.** Unknowingly, 53 million Americans drink tap water that is polluted by feces, radiation, or other contaminants. Half of all Americans drink water that has been *used* at least once before.

10. **Your Mouth.** A visit to your dentist could be deadly—unless you know what to look out for.

11. **Cleansing Your Liver and Blood.** Our liver is the primary filter of our body. Over time we so abuse it and so overtax it that illness is the inevitable result. Our blood is filled with many impurities including everything from an overabundance of artificial fats to toxic heavy metals. These must be removed for optimum health.

12. **The Immune System.** In many ways, your immune system is the most awesome system in your body, easily rivaling your brain in terms of complexity, subtlety, and *self-awareness.* And yet, we seem to do everything in our power to destroy it. For example, just one can of soda pop can depress your immune system by some 50% for as long as six hours. There is no chance for good health, or the elimination of disease, until your immune system has been optimized.

13. **The Thought That Kills.** What we think (and how we think) does absolutely (and unequivocally) affect our health. Or as Dr. John Christopher was fond of saying, "Most people need a colonic between the ears."

14. **Exercise.** It does everything from improving the health of the heart to building up your bones and speeding up the elimination of toxins from your body. The bottom line is that you must "move or die."

15. **Energy.** All life is energy. Optimize that energy and you optimize your health. Charge your body with the right frequencies and you prevent disease.

16. **Cancer.** The incidence of cancer is soaring—up between 800% to 1,700%

in the last 100 years (depending on whose numbers you look at).

In the last chapter, once you've learned the hows, whys, and wherefores of health, we will cut to the chase. I will detail **specific recommendations on what you can do to build your Baseline of Health, day-by-day.** I will outline a step-by-step program (based on all that has been learned from the miracle doctors and from over 30 years of my own work in cutting edge nutritionals) for optimizing your health and eliminating disease from your body.

So with that in mind, let's look, step by step, at how we maximize our Personal Health Line.

Chapter 3

Intestinal Cleansing, Detoxification and Rebuilding

There is an old saying that "death begins in the colon." This is an oversimplification to be sure, but more accurate than not. In fact, **the road to health begins with intestinal cleansing and detoxification—no matter what the disease or problem.**

Unfortunately, most people confine their understanding of intestinal cleansing to its effect on fecal matter. And while it is true that cleansing programs do draw old fecal matter out of the colon, limiting the discussion to fecal matter misses the big picture.

Understand that what we have is essentially a continuous tube from the mouth to the anus, and each part of that tube has a specific function to perform. Among these are:

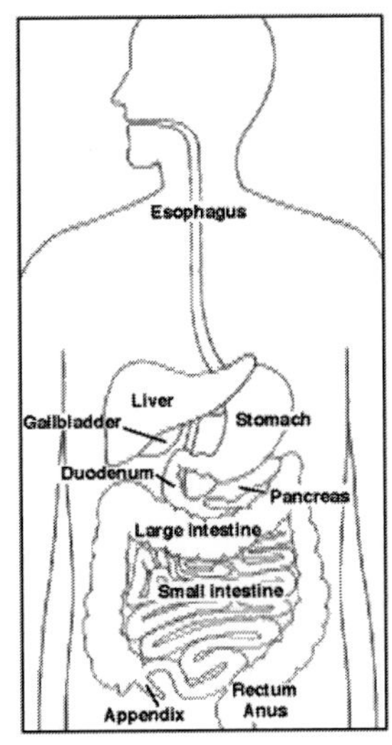

- Digestion of the food we eat.
- Transferring the nutritional value of that food into the body.
- Processing the waste from that food and eliminating it from the body.
- Serving as a drain pipe for waste produced as a result of metabolic functions within the body itself.
- Serving as a drain for toxic substances absorbed through our lungs and skin, etc.
- Functioning as a first line of defense in the body's immune system by identifying and eliminating viruses and unhealthy bacteria ingested with our food.

Any program of Intestinal Cleansing, Detoxification, and Rebuilding must address all of these aspects. Specifically, it must serve to:

- Remove all old fecal matter and waste from the colon (to clear the drain, if you will).
- Remove all the heavy metals and drug residues that have accumulated in the body as a result of having your drain plugged.
- Strengthen the colon muscle so that it works again.
- Repair any damage such as herniations and inflammations of the colon and small intestine.
- Eliminate the presence of polyps and other abnormal growths that have been allowed to flourish because of an unhealthy intestinal environment.
- Rebuild and replenish the various friendly bacteria cultures that ideally should line virtually every square inch of that tube—from mouth to anus.

The Problem

In 1985, between 60 and 70 million Americans were affected by digestive disorders. Today it's close to 100 million. **In fact, digestive disorders are responsible for over 50 million physician visits and more hospitalizations than any other category of medical problems in the United States today.** The total cost to the American public for all aspects of digestive disease is well over $100,000,000,000.00 per year.

What Digestive Diseases?

- Constipation and the attendant symptoms of self-toxification
- Diverticular disease (herniations of the colon)
- Hemorrhoids
- Irritable Bowel Syndrome
- Ulcerative Colitis
- Crohn's Disease
- Colon/Rectal Cancer
- Other Related Diseases

It is worth noting that many other diseases that at first glance appear to have no connection with the digestive tract have actually been related by many doctors to functional bowel disorder. These include: **Diabetes, Gall Stones, Kidney Stones, Gout, Hypertension, Varicose Veins, Rheumatoid Arthritis, Psoriasis, and Obesity.**

Parasites!

As if that were not enough, it has been estimated that as many as 80% of all Americans are afflicted with intestinal parasites.[1] Symptoms include nervousness, grinding of the teeth at night, aches and pains that move from place to place in the body, mimicked appendicitis, ulcers and various digestive pain, nausea or diarrhea, itching, acne, foul breath, furred tongue, jaundice, fatigue, menstrual irregularities, and insomnia.

Candida

And finally, more and more doctors are becoming aware of how endemic yeast infections such as *Candida Albicans* are. Symptoms include: chronic fatigue (especially after eating), depression, bloating, gas, cramps, chronic diarrhea or constipation, rectal itching, allergies, severe PMS, impotence, memory loss, severe mood swings, recurrent fungal infections (such as athlete's foot), extreme sensitivity to chemicals (perfumes, smoke, odors, etc.), and lightheadedness or drunkenness after minimal wine, beer, or sugar.

But It's Even Worse

The situation is serious. Diseases of the digestive system have reached an all-time high in the United States and are still on the rise. **The number one cancer among men and women combined is colon/rectal cancer.**

According to the *Merck Manual* (the medical industry's standard text for the diagnosis and treatment of disease), **the incidence of diverticulosis has increased dramatically over the last 40 years.** It has gone from 10% of the adult population over the age of 45 who had this disease (according to an early 1950s edition) to an astounding, "every person has many" in the 1992 edition. **In other words, virtually 100% of all American adults will eventually have diverticulosis of the large intestine if they live long enough.**

Why?

Our modern lifestyle has taken its toll on our digestive/elimination organs. Refined, processed, low-fiber foods, animal fats, a lack of exercise, and an ever increasing level of stress all contribute to our current gastrointestinal health crisis.

---

[1]Many health professionals would dispute this number, calling it far too high. And if you limit your discussion of parasites to things such as tape worms and Chinese liver flukes, they are correct. But the fact is, as soon as you open up to the true nature of the problem and begin including the lesser known, but far more prevalent, parasites such as Demodex human and Fasciolosis buskii, the 80% figure begins to fall into line. And then if you include *E. coli* and *Candida* overgrowths (both of which fit the dictionary definition of a parasite: any organism that grows and feeds in another while contributing nothing in return), then the 80% figure is decidedly conservative.

Consider that a sluggish bowel can retain pounds of old toxic and poisonous fecal matter (10–20 pounds is not unusual, and up to 65 pounds has actually been reported). Many times the real cause behind sickness and disease is this retention and reabsorption of built-up toxic waste.

There has been a great misconception among the public and most medical professionals about how often a normal healthy person should move their bowels. For years, doctors have thought that anywhere between one bowel movement a day and one a week was normal. What we have learned is that it is normal, *and necessary,* to have one bowel movement a day for each major meal you eat. (If you eat three meals, you should have three bowel movements the next day.)

Toxic Lymph

Think for a moment, if you will, of your colon as your body's drain pipe—the drain that removes waste from your body. If the drain is clogged, not only will waste not be eliminated, but when you flush the toilet, the drain backs up and spills over.

And that's exactly the point which leads us to a discussion of waste removal from the body and the lymph system.

The lymph vessels comprise a network of capillaries which filter blood impurities; they contain a clear, colorless fluid (lymph). Lymph passes from capillaries to lymph vessels and flows through lymph nodes that are located along the course of these vessels. Cells of the lymph nodes phagocytize, or ingest, such impurities as bacteria, old red blood cells, and toxic and cellular waste. Lymph fluid can also collect other impurities such as heavy metals and pesticides and drug residues stored in bodily tissue. Once loaded with toxic waste, the compromised lymph must exit your body.

What can't be eliminated in your urine must pass out through your colon. What do you think happens to all this waste if the plumbing is plugged or sluggish? Is it any wonder we get sick and keep on getting sicker?

Probiotics

We're going to be discussing probiotics in detail in the next chapter, but for now, it's worth noting their importance in maintaining not only intestinal health, but overall health. Our intestinal tract contains hundreds of billions of bacteria—all microscopic in size—and yet, because of their sheer numbers, their total weight is close to 3 ½ pounds in the average adult. Approximately ⅓ of the dry weight of our fecal matter is composed of bacteria—living and dead, harmful and beneficial. A major indicator of the state of our health, both intestinal and overall, is in the composition of those bacteria.

What Can Be Done?

Any program designed to clean, detoxify, and rebuild the colon needs to address several key areas. The program must:

- Help bring the colon back to life by stimulating the muscle movement of the colon.
- Encourage matter to move forward through the system.
- Halt putrefaction.
- Draw old fecal matter off the walls of the colon and out of any bowel pockets.
- Disinfect.
- Draw out poisons and toxins.
- Help leach out heavy metals such as mercury and lead.
- Remove chemicals and drug residues.
- Even remove radioactive material such as Strontium 90.
- Soothe and promote the healing of the mucous membrane lining of the entire digestive tract.
- Help stimulate the body to begin the healing and repair of herniated areas.
- Increase the flow of bile to help clean the gall bladder, bile ducts, and liver.
- Promote healthy intestinal flora.
- Destroy and expel parasites.
- Destroy *Candida albicans* overgrowth.
- Maintain regularity.
- Decrease straining.
- Speed up the transit time of feces through the large intestine.
- Promote the growth of beneficial bacteria colonies in the intestinal tract.

Once you look at the requirements of a good intestinal program, it's easy to see that no one formula or magic pill can accomplish it all.

Summary

The foundation of any health or healing program must begin with the intestinal tract—not necessarily because it is inherently more important than any other system or organ in the body, but because it's the area of the body upon which we focus our greatest abuse, and because it impacts virtually every other system in the body. This point is so important that it's worth reviewing the core issues that we've covered in this chapter.

1. The colon is the main elimination channel of the body. It is the means by which we eliminate the toxic waste of the digestive process, including massive amounts of *E. coli* bacteria and parasite larvae. If that waste hangs around longer than necessary, its impact on the body is profound. And yet, because of dietary and health habits, **the average American stores, on average, between 10–20 pounds of old (sometimes decades old) fecal matter in their colons.** I personally know of people who, while on a colon cleansing program, have passed the coins they had swallowed, or the multicolored waxes of the crayons they had eaten when they were children, over 50 years ago.

2. The liver is the main detoxifying organ of the body. It filters out dangerous drug residues and poisons from the blood and passes them out of the body—through the colon via the bile duct. Plug the colon and it's like flushing a toilet plugged with toilet paper; everything backs up. The net result is sickness and disease. **The important point to remember here is that you can't even begin to cleanse and repair the other systems in the body until you clean out the colon so that the toxic material will have a clean path out of the body**.

3. Physically, the colon is not designed to store large amounts of old fecal matter. There just isn't room for it. If you have 10, 20, 30 pounds of extra garbage in there, there's only one thing that can happen; the colon must distend and expand. This causes the walls of the colon to thin out (like blowing up a balloon more and more). As the walls extend out, they press on and compress other organs in the abdominal cavity.

4. Old fecal matter is an ideal breeding ground for harmful bacteria and dangerous parasites.

5. Intestinal flora are an essential part of health. If you eat foods laced with antibiotics and drink water with chlorine in it, you eliminate virtually all beneficial bacteria—providing an absolutely open environment for the proliferation of harmful bacteria, such as *E. coli.*

6. Your intestinal tract is the source of all nutrient access to your body. If it isn't working properly, you have two major problems.
   - First, you have a hard time digesting food properly—breaking it down sufficiently so that your body can use it.
   - And then, even if you can digest it properly, if the intestinal wall is covered with hardened waste and colonies of hostile bacteria/flora, you'll end up absorbing only a fraction of the nutritional value of the food you eat.

The bottom line is that any program we design to improve our health or to eliminate disease from our bodies must begin with Intestinal Cleansing, Detoxification, and Rebuilding. It is the "sine qua non"[1] of health.

General Recommendations

What is required is a four-pronged approach.

- A probiotic formula to promote the growth of beneficial bacteria colonies in the intestinal tract.
- A good source of **fiber** to compensate for all of the fiberless processed foods, meat, and dairy that we eat.
  - The best single source of fiber in the world is ground organic flaxseed meal. One and a half tablespoons twice a day with juice will keep you regular and also provide you with the best single source of Omega-3 oils in the world. In addition, the sulfur-rich proteins present in the seeds work hand in hand with the Omega-3 oils to literally reverse mutated cells and cancer in the body.
- For many people, a good probiotic formula alone will serve to wake up their colon and get it working again. Most people, however will need a stimulating **herbal colon-activator** formula that provides both cleansing and healing to the entire gastrointestinal system (at least until their colons rebuild).
  - Look for a formula that contains all organic herbs such as: Cape Aloe, Senna, Cascara Sagrada, Barberry Rootbark, Ginger Root, African Bird Pepper, and Fennel.
  - This formula will serve as an intestinal detoxifier to loosen and draw out old fecal matter, waste, and toxins. It will stimulate peristalsis (the muscular movement of the colon). It will also halt putrefaction, disinfect, and soothe and heal the mucous membrane lining of your entire digestive tract. It will also help improve digestion, relieve gas and cramps, increase the flow of bile (which in turn cleans the gall bladder, bile ducts, and liver), destroy *Candida albicans* overgrowth, and promote a healthy intestinal flora, destroy and expel intestinal parasites, and increase gastrointestinal circulation.
- Periodically (approximately every 3 months), you will need a **strong purifier and intestinal vacuum** to help draw old fecal matter off the walls of your colon and out of any bowel pockets and to also draw out poisons, toxins, heavy metals (such as mercury and lead), and even remove radioactive material such as Strontium 90 from your body. Such a formula will also remove over 2,000 known drug residues.

---

[1]Literally, "Without which, there is not."

- Look for a formula that contains all organic herbs such as: Apple Fruit Pectin, pharmaceutical grade Montmorillonite Clay, Slippery Elm Inner Bark, Marshmallow Root, Fennel Seed, Activated Willow Charcoal, and psyllium seeds and husks.
- The natural mucilaginous properties of this formula will soften old hardened fecal matter for easy removal and also make it an excellent remedy for any inflammation or irritation in the stomach and intestines. This formula is helpful in irritable bowel syndrome, diverticular disease, and hemorrhoids.
- And on top of everything else, this formula will eliminate the effects of food poisoning or stomach flu in 20–40 minutes!

Regular use of this four-part program will help keep your body in optimal health and vitality for as long as you live.

CHAPTER 4

THE PROBIOTIC MIRACLE

AN ARMY OF BILLIONS

When you were born, your intestines were virtually sterile, free of microorganisms. Almost immediately, however, bacteria, both friendly and harmful, fought for dominance.[1] If you were breast fed, somewhere between days four and seven after you were born, the beneficial bacteria won the battle and staked their claim to virtually every square inch of your digestive tract—from your mouth to your anus.[2] (Researchers now realize that one of the chief reasons breast-fed babies get so many fewer infections than formula-fed babies is that mother's milk tends to promote superior growth of beneficial bacteria in the gastrointestinal tract, whereas store-bought formulas have little such beneficial effect.) Anyway, the net result is that in a breast-fed baby, beneficial bacteria (such as bifidobacteria) control over 90% of the intestinal tract. These microorganisms, in turn, produce a large amount of essential byproducts in the intestines, which act as a barrier to the growth of dangerous pathogenic microbes that can cause disease and infection.

When you are healthy, over 100 trillion microorganisms from some 400 different species flourish in your intestinal tract, aiding in digestion, absorption, and the production of significant amounts of B vitamins and enzymes. But even more importantly, they cover virtually every square inch of available surface space in your large and small intestines, thus crowding out all harmful bacteria—allowing them no place to gain a foothold.

Unfortunately, the levels of beneficial bacteria decline dramatically as the human body ages. Some of the reasons for this decline include:

- Over time, the colonies of friendly bacteria just naturally age and lose their vitality.
- Disruptions and changes in the acid/alkaline balance of the bowels can play a major role in reducing the growth of beneficial bacteria. In addition, these

---

[1]It's a battle that's never totally won; the harmful bacteria are never completely eliminated. But in a healthy body, the bad guys never get a chance to gain a foothold—to colonize—to reproduce exponentially. One of the problems, of course, is that every second of every single day, we are constantly being exposed to billions and billions of potentially harmful microorganisms with every breath we take or bit of food that we swallow or swig of water that we drink.

[2]The same battle is fought in the vaginal tract, the nasal cavities, and in the mouth. Just as a note, there are some 40 different types of bacteria resident in a healthy mouth alone.

changes tend to favor the growth of harmful viral and fungal organisms as well as putrefactive, disease-causing bacteria.

- Non-steroidal anti-inflammatory drugs (NSAIDS) like Advil, Motrin, Midol, etc. are destructive to intestinal flora.
- Chlorine in the drinking water not only serves to kill bacteria in the water; it is equally devastating to the colonies of beneficial bacteria living in the intestines.
- Radiation and chemotherapy are devastating to your inner bacterial environment.
- Virtually all meat, chicken, and dairy that you eat (other than organic) is loaded with antibiotics, which destroy **all** of the beneficial bacteria in your gastrointestinal tract.
- A diet high in meats and fats, because they take so long to break down in the human body, promotes the growth of the harmful, putrefying bacteria.
- Constipation, of course, allows harmful bacteria to hang around longer, which allows them to proliferate.
- Cigarettes, alcohol, and stress are also major culprits, as are some antibiotic herbs, such as goldenseal (if taken in sufficient quantity).
- And if you've ever been subjected to a round of "medicinal" antibiotics, you can kiss your beneficial bacteria goodbye. The problem is that antibiotics indiscriminately destroy both bad and **good** bacteria, allowing virulent, mutant strains of harmful microorganisms to emerge and run rampant inside the body.[1].

A properly functioning intestinal tract is one of your body's first lines of defense against invaders. In a healthy colon there are, on average, anywhere from 100 billion to 100 trillion **beneficial** bacteria per milliliter (about $\frac{1}{5}$ of a teaspoon) that literally consume harmful bacteria and other invaders. In the typical American, because of poor diet and neglect of the colon, the beneficial bacteria count may be as low as four or five per milliliter. Just compare 100 trillion to four, and you'll have an understanding of the scope of the problem. Many researchers now believe that declining levels of friendly bacteria in the intestinal tract may actually mark the onset of chronic degenerative disease. The benefits of a probiotically optimized intestinal tract include:

- Lowered cholesterol
- Inhibition of cancer

---

[1]Antibiotics (both medicinal and in our food supply) are the #1 culprit in the overgrowth of **harmful** pathogens in the gastrointestinal tract (a condition called dysbiosis) that may be at the root of many autoimmune disorders and certain cancers.

- Protection against food poisoning
- Protection against stomach ulcers
- Protection against lactose intolerance and casein intolerance
- Enhanced immunity
- Protection against many harmful bacteria, viruses, and fungi
- Protection against candida overgrowth and vaginal yeast infections
- Prevention and correction of constipation and diarrhea, ileitis and colitis, irritable bowel syndrome, and a whole range of other digestive tract dysfunctions
- Improvement in the health and appearance of the skin
- Better nutrition from improved absorption and the internal generation of B vitamins.
- Protection against vaginosis and yeast infections

Summary

There can be no true health or recovery from disease unless you have colonies of over 100 trillion beneficial microorganisms flourishing in your intestinal tract, aiding in digestion, absorption, the production of significant amounts of vitamins and enzymes, and working to crowd out all harmful bacteria—allowing them no place to gain a foothold. **Supplementation with a good probiotic is mandatory to raise your baseline of health.**

General Recommendations

- A good probiotic formula is absolutely essential for long-term intestinal health and long-term parasite control. When choosing a probiotic, look for the following characteristics:
  - Not all strains of beneficial bacteria are created equal. For each type of bacteria, there are recognized super strains. Choose a formula that uses only recognized super strains of beneficial bacteria. They will be identified as such on the label or in the company literature. If the strains are not identified, don't buy it.
  - Make sure the formula you choose was developed using full-culture processing so that the beneficial bacteria **and its all-important supernatant** are kept together. The supernatant, which is the medium the culture was grown in, contains a multitude of beneficial byproducts of the growth process, including vitamins, enzymes, antidants, and immune stimulators.

- Then there's the question of how many live microorganisms are left in your formula when you actually use it. Pick up any probiotic formula, look at the label, and you'll see something like: "Contains 13 billion live organisms per capsule at time of manufacture." And that's the problem: "at time of manufacture." The die-off rate can be astounding. Most formulas will experience a die-off approaching log-3 (or down to a paltry 13 million) within just 60 days of manufacture.[1] Heat and moisture accelerate the process, which is why most manufacturers recommend that both you and the store in which you bought your formula keep your probiotic supply refrigerated.

- There are many beneficial bacteria that can be contained in a good probiotic, but two are preeminent. Look for a formula based on these two:
  - *L. acidophilus* resides primarily in the small intestine[2] and produces a number of powerful antimicrobial compounds in the gut (including acidolin, acidolphilin, lactocidin, and bacteriocin). These compounds can inhibit the growth and toxin producing capabilities of some 23 known disease-causing pathogens (including campylobacter, listeria, and staphylococci), as well as reduce tumor growth and effectively neutralize or inhibit carcinogenic substances. There are three recognized super strains of acidophilus: DDS, NAS, and BT1386. You will find DDS and NAS in most of the better formulas, but my personal preference is for BT1386. It has an extremely high potential for attachment to the epithelial cells that line the intestine; it's a high producer of hydrogen peroxide, which kills pathogenic bacteria; and, of the three strains, it's the only one capable of utilizing glycogen to survive and flourish, which means it can thrive in the urinary tract, where it produces lactic acid to inhibit the growth of pathogens. This is particularly important to women to help prevent a whole range of vaginal infections.
  - Many researchers believe that declining levels of *bifidobacteria* in the large intestine actually mark the eventual onset of chronic degenerative disease. *Bifidobacteria* benefit the body in a number of ways. They (1) consume old fecal matter; (2) have the ability to remove cancer-forming elements, or the enzymes which lead to their formation; (3) protect against the formation of liver, colon, and mammary gland tumors. And in addition to all of that, (4) *bifidobacteria* are substantial producers of a range of important B vitamins.

- More is not always better. Too many beneficial bacteria in one formula may find the bacteria competing with each other before they can establish themselves in

---

[1]There is a new process called LiveBac®, which significantly retards the rate of die-off. Look for formulas that make use of this process.

[2]It's also important to note that L. acidophilus is the primary beneficial bacteria in the vaginal tract. When the presence of the acidophilus is compromised, this allows the bad guys such as *Gardnerella vaginalis* or *E. coli* or *Chlamydia* to take over.

separate areas of the intestinal tract. On the other hand, there are several other bacteria that are extremely beneficial in any probiotic formula.

- *L. salivarius* helps digest foods in the intestinal tract and makes vital nutrients more assimilable. It also works to eat away encrusted fecal matter throughout the entire colon; it helps repair the intestinal tract by providing needed enzymes and essential nutrients; and it adheres to the intestinal wall, thereby forming a living matrix that helps protect the mucosal lining.
- *L. rhamnosus* is a powerful immune stimulator. It can increase the natural killing activity of spleen cells, which may help to prevent tumor formation. It boosts the ability of the body to destroy foreign invaders and other harmful matter by three times normal activity, and has been shown to increase circulating antibody levels by six to eight times.
- *L. plantarum* has the ability to eliminate thousands of species of pathogenic bacteria. It also has extremely high adherence potential for epithelial tissue and seems to favor colonizing the same areas of the intestinal tract that *E. coli* prefers—in effect, serving to crowd *E. coli* out of the body. At one time, plantarum was a major part of our diets (found in sourdough bread, sauerkraut, etc.), but is now virtually nowhere to be found.
- Other important friendly bacteria you might find in a good formula include: *Streptococcus thermophilus, L. bulgaricus,* and *L. casei.*
- Much has been written about the properties of the soil-based bacteria such as: *Bacillus subtilis, L. sporogenes,* and *B. laterosporus.* For many people, they can produce a powerful boost to the immune system. **But, in certain circumstances, they may become toxic.** It's hard to argue with the great results that many people have had using formulations that contain these cultures. On the other hand, it's possible to get all of the same results using only the "safer" cultures that I've mentioned above.
- Note: a good probiotic formulation will usually contain fructo-oligosaccharides (FOS) which help promote the growth of beneficial bacteria.[1]
- One final note: start slowly. **When you first start using a probiotic supplement, there is a good chance that you will precipitate a die-off of bad bacteria in your intestinal tract.** This can lead to excessive gas and stomach rumblings and cramping for 10-21 days. Start with one capsule (or even half) for several days. Build up slowly to the recommended dosage for your particular supplement.

- Eating yogurt (unless you make your own) does not really help. First, the bacteria used to make most yogurt (*L. bulgaricus* and *S. thermophilus*) are not the key beneficial bacteria, although they are indeed helpful. (Some brands throw a small amount of acidophilus in after the fact—just so they can put it on the

---

[1]For some of these bacteria, such as the Bifidus, FOS can increase their effectiveness by a factor of 1,000 times or more!!

label). Even more important, though, **much of the yogurt that you buy in the store is now pasteurized after** it is made. Pasteurization **before** the yogurt culture is introduced is essential to the making of yogurt; but **pasteurization after the culture has been allowed to grow is done merely to increase shelf life and totally destroys all the benefits inherent in the yogurt.**

- A diet high in complex carbohydrates such as fruits, grains, and vegetables promotes the growth of bifidobacteria in the large intestine.
- And of course, drinking chlorinated water, or eating meats or dairy produced with antibiotics, totally defeats any program you're on.

Chapter 5

Enzymes = Life

Anyone who has any understanding of health has got to be taking enzyme supplements with every single meal they eat. Unfortunately, most people think of enzymes (if they think of them at all) as necessary only if they have some kind of digestive problem. And, yes, it's true that people suffering from digestive problems, hiatal hernias, ulcers, and the like, have benefited greatly from using enzyme supplements. But if that's all you think enzymes are for, you've missed the point. Dr. Howell, in his book on enzyme nutrition, puts it quite clearly when he says that **a person's life span is directly related to the exhaustion of their enzyme potential. And the use of food enzymes decreases that rate of exhaustion, and thus, results in a longer, healthier, and more vital life.**

Now that pretty much says it all. But just to drive the point home, let's go into the enzyme story in a little more detail.

The Enzyme Story

Enzymes are proteins that facilitate chemical reactions in living organisms. In fact, they are **required** for every single chemical action that takes place in your body. All of your tissues, muscles, bones, organs, and cells are run by enzymes.

Your digestive system, immune system, blood stream, liver, kidneys, spleen, and pancreas, as well as your ability to see, think, feel, and breathe, (in fact, the very functioning of each and every cell in your body) all depend on enzymes. All of the minerals and vitamins you eat and all of the hormones your body produces need enzymes in order to work properly. In fact, every single metabolic function in your body is governed by enzymes. Your stamina, your energy level, your ability to utilize vitamins and minerals, your immune system—all governed by enzymes.

But where do enzymes come from? As it happens, they are produced both internally (in every cell in your body, but most notably in the pancreas and the other endocrine glands), and they are present in all of the **raw** foods that we eat. At birth, we are endowed with a certain potential for manufacturing enzymes in our bodies, an enzyme "reserve," if you will. Nature intended that we continually replenish that reserve through proper nutrition and eating habits. Unfortunately, that just doesn't happen. Let's take a look at why.

Most people believe that when you eat a meal it drops into a pool of stomach acid, where it's broken down, then goes into the small intestine to have nutrients taken out, and then into the colon to be passed out of the body—if you're lucky. Not quite.

What nature intended is that you eat enzyme rich foods and chew your food properly. If you did that, the food would enter the stomach laced with digestive enzymes. These enzymes would then "predigest" your food for about an hour—actually breaking down as much as 75% of your meal.

After this period of "pre-digestion," hydrochloric acid is introduced. The acid inactivates all of the food-based enzymes, but begins its own function of breaking down what is left of the meal. Eventually, this nutrient-rich food concentrate moves on into the small intestine. Once this concentrate enters the small intestine, the acid is neutralized and the pancreas reintroduces digestive enzymes to the process. As digestion is completed, nutrients are passed through the intestinal wall and into the blood stream.

That's what nature intended. Unfortunately, most of us don't live our lives as nature intended!

Processing and cooking destroy enzymes in food. **(Man is the only animal that cooks his food.)** In fact, any sustained heat of approximately 118°–129° F destroys virtually all enzymes. This means that, for most of us, the food entering our stomachs is severely enzyme deficient. (Actually, there are some enzymes present from our saliva. The amount, however, is minuscule since we only chew our food about 25% as much as is required.) The result is that most of our meals enter our stomachs woefully devoid of enzymes.

The food then sits there for an hour, like a heavy lump, with very little predigestion taking place. Even after the stomach acid has done its work, the meal enters the small intestine largely undigested.

At this point, the pancreas and the other organs of the endocrine system are put under tremendous stress since they have to draw reserves from the entire body in order to produce massive amounts of the proper enzymes. **The less digestion that takes place before food reaches the small intestine, the greater the stress placed on the endocrine systems. Recent studies have shown that virtually 100% of all Americans have an enlarged pancreas by the time they are 40.** Is it any wonder that the incidence of diabetes is exploding in the developed world?[1]

There is also major research showing that enzyme deficient diets contribute to a pathological enlargement of the pituitary gland. (That's the gland that regulates all the other glands in the body.) And there is research showing that almost 100% of people over 50 who die from "accidental" causes have defective pituitary glands.

The bottom line is that regular supplementation with digestive enzymes takes

---

[1]The ever increasing intake of refined carbohydrates such as sugar is also a major contributing factor.

stress off the pancreas (and the entire body) by providing the enzymes required for digestion. **In other words, digestive enzyme supplements may just be one of the best insurance policies you can give your body so you can enjoy a long and healthy life.**

All of what you've just read should be convincing; but just in case it's not, let me give you three real-world examples of the power of digestive enzymes in action.

- F. M. Pottenger, M.D., and D. G. Simonsen conducted a series of studies to determine what, if any, impact cooked food had on health. They put two groups of cats on controlled diets, identical except that in one group the food was raw, and in the second group the food was cooked. The results were astounding. The group on raw food maintained normal good health throughout the experiments and showed no sign of degenerative diseases, but the group on cooked meat showed an astonishing breakdown of health in all the animals, including:
  - Incomplete development of the skull and other bones
  - Bowed legs
  - Rickets
  - Curvature of the spine
  - Paralysis of the legs
  - Seizures
  - Convulsions
  - Thyroid abscesses
  - Cyanosis of the liver and kidneys
  - Enlarged colon
  - Degeneration of motor nerves throughout the brain and spine
  - **And by the third generation, this group could not reproduce**
- Studies done with laboratory rats have shown that rats eating raw foods live about 30% longer than rats eating diets devoid of enzymes.
- Then there's the fact that the classic Eskimo diet consists of 80% saturated fat? That's 80% saturated fat (primarily from raw fat and raw meat)! And yet, in a study of 3,000 of these people, not one of them had high cholesterol, heart disease, arteriosclerosis, or high blood pressure. And only one of the 3,000 was even slightly overweight.

Now don't get me wrong, I am not advocating that you live on seal blubber like the Eskimos and raw meat like the Pottenger cats. But, can there be any doubt in your mind that live enzymes in your diet make a dramatic difference in your overall health and longevity?

But There's Even More

Pancreatic enzymes are part of a substance called **pancreatin** (or pancreas juice) produced in the pancreas. This complex includes the enzymes protease, amylase, and lipase and is released both into the intestines **and the bloodstream.**

In the intestines, pancreatin works to help digest the proteins, carbohydrates, and starches of our meals. Supplementation with digestive enzymes **along with a meal** helps share the workload of your body's own pancreatic enzymes and can aid in digestion. But what happens if you take enzymes **between meals?**

As mentioned earlier, pancreatic enzymes are not only released into the small intestine, but also directly into the bloodstream. Why?

Protein molecules that are only partially digested in the small intestine are absorbed into the bloodstream. Once in the bloodstream, the immune system treats them as invaders provoking an immune reaction. Antibodies couple with these foreign protein invaders to form circulating immune complexes (CIC's). In a healthy person, these CIC's may be neutralized in the lymphatic system. But if the immune system is in any way compromised, CIC's accumulate in the blood, where they initiate an "allergic" reaction. As the number of CIC's builds, the kidneys max out and can no longer excrete all of them, so they begin to accumulate in the body's soft tissues, causing inflammation.

It is here that the pancreatic enzymes in our bloodstream come into play. Pancreatic enzymes are able to break down CIC's so that they can pass through the kidneys for excretion.

What does that mean for supplemental enzymes? Well, if enzymes are taken between meals, the body doesn't need the enzymes for digesting food, so they make their way directly into the bloodstream to aid in the elimination of CIC's.

But it gets even better. Because of their ability to digest foreign proteins, pancreatic enzymes (both those produced in the body and those absorbed into the bloodstream from your supplement) work to clear out infecting organisms such as viruses, scar tissue, and the products of inflammation. For this reason, pancreatic enzymes are frequently used by Naturopaths to treat a variety of conditions, including lung infections, tooth infections, bone fractures, and as a body strengthener before surgery. Specifically, pancreatic enzymes have been used by many healers to aid in a variety of disease conditions, including inflammation, viral disease, multiple sclerosis, and cancer.

Conclusion

As Dr. Howell said: **a person's life span is directly related to the exhaustion of their enzyme potential. And the use of food enzymes decreases that rate of exhaustion, and thus, results in a longer, healthier, and more vital life.** The question for you, then, is how could you not be insisting that everyone you know and love use enzymes every time they eat? How could you not be using them every time you yourself eat? This is a no brainer. In addition to a longer, healthier, and more vital life, you will also experience a number of short-term benefits, including:

- A significant reduction in indigestion and heartburn problems resulting from too much acid in the stomach.
- Since complex carbohydrates are now being substantially digested before they enter the intestinal tract, you should experience relief from gas and bloating.[1]
- Look for improved digestion of dairy products.
- Diminished food allergies due to more complete protein digestion.
- Since the digestion of enzyme deficient food is an extremely energy consuming task, within a few days of enzyme supplementation you should notice:
    - An increase in energy levels.
    - Relief from hiatal hernias.
    - Relief from ulcers.[2]

AN EXPERIMENT

There is a fun experiment you can perform (that will work with any good digestive enzyme formula) which will actually let you see the benefit of enzyme supplementation in just a few minutes.

1. Make two bowls of **instant** oatmeal.
2. Crush (or mix) the contents of a couple of digestive enzyme capsules into just one of the bowls of oatmeal.
3. Wait 45 minutes.

---

[1]Some people may actually notice an increase in activity for several days as their digestive systems come alive.

[2]Digestive enzymes help with ulcers in two ways. First, they help digest so much of your meal during the 40–60 minutes of predigestion that your body requires less acid in the actual digestion phase. This means that taking digestive enzymes will help lower the levels of acid in your stomach. (Those who suffer from chronic low levels of acid need not worry. Digestive enzyme supplements help here, too, by breaking down so much food in the predigestion phase that less acid is actually required. And over time, decreased demand results in increased reserve capability.)

Second, protease will begin breaking down the protective coating of the H. Pylori bacteria responsible for so many ulcers. In other words, it will actually begin to digest it. This is the prime reason digestive enzyme supplements are so helpful for those who have ulcers.

A cautionary note. There is one concern when using digestive enzymes with ulcers—and that's if you have a severe existing ulcer. What happens is that the protease can actually begin to digest severely damaged stomach lining tissue. This can cause noticeable discomfort for several days. To avoid this discomfort, if you have a severe ulcer, start with small amounts of the supplement with your meals and build up slowly.

4. Now check. If the formula you are using is any good, there should be a pronounced difference in the two bowls. The untreated bowl should be as expected: a congealed, lumpy, stick-to-your-ribs consistency. The bowl with the enzymes, however, will look quite different. It will be "digested" and have the consistency of watery gruel. Which oatmeal would you rather have work through your body: the one that's stuck to the bowl like cement, or the enzyme bowl that's predigested? Which oatmeal do you think is less stressful to digest?

Summary

As I mentioned earlier, a person's life span is directly related to the exhaustion of their enzyme potential. And the use of food enzymes decreases that rate of exhaustion, and thus, results in a longer, healthier, and more vital life. **At a minimum, you must use a good enzyme supplement with each and every meal you eat—particularly any meal that contains either processed or cooked food.**

General Recommendations

- But which enzymes should you use? The fact is you'll benefit from any good vegetarian-based enzyme supplement. But look for one that contains several protein digestors such as **Protease** and **Papain** (to aid in the digestion of protein), **Amylase** (for the digestion of starches and carbohydrates), **Lipase** and **Bromelain** (to digest fats), **Cellulase** (invaluable in breaking down fiber cellulose into smaller units), and **Lactase** (which works in the digestion of dairy products).

- You can also identify good enzyme supplements by the inclusion of coenzyme factors, which serve to substantially increase the efficacy of the supplement. The standard factors you will find include probiotics (such as bifidus), chelated minerals, algae (such as spirulina and chlorella), and ionic minerals.
  - Probiotics are effective, but as I mentioned in the last chapter, they are subject to a high die-off rate, which means practically no probiotic activity is left by the time you take your enzyme supplement.
  - As for chelated minerals, they too are effective, but I have a fundamental problem with chelated minerals. I believe that chelation is a way to trick the body into absorbing minerals that are in a form your body has a hard time assimilating—unlike the biologically transformed minerals found in plants.
  - Which leaves algae and ionic minerals as the best coenzyme factor to use in an enzyme supplement.

- Note: Another ingredient you will sometimes find in enzyme formulations is Betaine HCL. Many people, particularly as they get older, produce insufficient stomach acid for proper digestion. For these people, supplementation with Betaine HCL makes sense, but not in an enzyme formula. As we previously discussed, many of the digestive enzymes are neutralized in an acid environment—which is why they do most of their work in that 40–60-minute period of predigestion that takes place after eating, before stomach acid is released. If you take Betaine, it's best to take it as a separate supplement 40–60 minutes after eating.
- Another ingredient that you may find in some enzyme formulas is mastic gum. Mastic, which is widely used in Mediterranean cooking as a sweetening agent, offers no direct enzymatic benefits, but it nevertheless offers a couple of interesting health benefits.
    - First, studies now indicate that mastic renders H. pylori (the stomach ulcer bacteria) vulnerable to your body's immune system.
    - Mastic also enhances your body's ability to regenerate the epithelial cells of your gastrointestinal lining.
    - The net result is that mastic can help prevent and relieve a number of digestive disorders, including heartburn, gas, bloating, dyspepsia, and nausea.
    - Should you use a formula that contains mastic? It's pretty much a neutral call. The mastic definitely provides some important digestive benefits (particularly if you suffer from stomach ulcers); however, for every milligram of mastic in your formula, that's one milligram less of enzymes present.
- A couple of times a week at night (or more often if you think of it), before bed, take your enzyme supplement on an empty stomach.
- As when taking a probiotic supplement, start slowly. In order to avoid excessive intestinal agitation and discomfort,[1] start by using the lowest possible dosage of your enzyme supplement for the first few days. Then gradually build up your dosage to the recommended amount.

[1]Gas, bloating, diarrhea, and constipation are all possible when first starting supplementation with enzymes. Stick with it. After about three weeks, your body settles down and you can begin to receive all of the benefits with no downside.

Chapter 6

Diet, the Slow Killer

Once, you've cleaned out and repaired your food processing and waste removal system, you're ready to begin the process of rebuilding your body. Keep in mind that your body is rebuilding itself all the time. The actual life cycle of a blood cell, for example, is approximately four months. That means you end up replacing your entire blood supply every 120 days. The question is what will determine the quality of that blood? What are you going to be building that new blood from—Cocoa Puffs and beer?

Understand, it's not only your blood, but every cell and organ in your body that's being replaced. For the most part, you get an entirely new body every seven years. It doesn't take a genius to realize that **the better your nutrition, the better "quality" of your new body.**

Unfortunately, it's not so simple. Any attempt to optimize the nutrition we take into our bodies must address five key problem areas.

The Five Problem Areas

1. The Question of Meat
2. Milk. It Doesn't Necessarily Do a Body Good
3. Plastic Fats
4. Refined to Death
5. What's the Big Deal about Organic (which will be covered in Chapter 7)

1. The Question of Meat

Probably no topic has been more discussed (and is more confusing) than what constitutes the optimum diet. There's the:

- Caveman diet
- The Blood-type diet
- The Hi-carbo diet
- The Low-carbo diet

- The High-protein diet
- The Low-protein diet
- The Steak Lover's diet
- The Vegetarian diet
- The Vegan (or pure vegetarian) diet
- The Hollywood diet
- The Scarsdale diet
- The Twinkie diet
- etc.

Heck, I'm getting confused just writing them down. So let's step back, take an objective view of the situation, and do a little reality check.

Let's begin by cutting through all of the nonsense and just taking a look at what kinds of food our bodies were designed to handle—then figure out what that means for us today. And the best way to do that is by first identifying the key characteristics of our "eating and digestive" systems, then seeing which animals we match up with and what they eat. The key "indicators" that we're going to look at are:

- The teeth
- The stomach
- The length of the digestive tract

The Human Eating Machine

- Teeth
  - All of our teeth are nearly of the same height. Our canines are projected only a small amount, and our molars are broad-topped
- Stomach
  - The human stomach is slightly elongated, approximating the shape of a kidney bean
- Digestive tract
  - The average adult has a digestive tract (measured from mouth to anus) of about 30–33 feet long. This means that the ratio of the length of a person's digestive tract as compared to their height (also measured from mouth to anus) is approximately 10–12 times the length of their body.

Carnivores, the Meat Eaters: Lions, Tigers, Etc.

The first thing you notice about carnivores is that their teeth are nothing like those found in humans. They have huge canines for striking and seizing prey, pointed incisors for removing meat from bones, and molars and premolars with cusps for shredding muscle fiber. In carnivores, the teeth of the upper jaw slide past the outside of the lower jaw so that prey is caught in a vicelike grip. **In general, carnivores don't chew much; mostly, they just tear chunks off and swallow them whole.**

An examination of the carnivore intestinal tract reveals a short (relative to the length of their body) bowel for fast transit of waste out of the body.[1] (The actual length of the carnivore bowel is approximately 3 to 5 times the length of the body—measured from mouth to anus—**a ratio less than half that found in humans.)**

Most of the digestive process occurs in the carnivore's stomach (which is a round, sack-shaped, simple structure with a very high concentration of acid salts for digesting animal muscle and bone). **Food usually remains for days at a time in a carnivore's stomach while it is digested (to a large extent) by enzymes present in the *raw* meat itself (a process called autolytic digestion).** In addition, carnivores are adapted to process huge amounts of food at a time (up to 25% of their body weight or more), then eat nothing for days at a time.

Again, this doesn't sound very much like us.

Herbivores, the Plant Eaters: Cows, Deer, Etc.

Herbivores have sharp chisel-shaped incisors for cutting, no upper incisors in some cases, and small incisor-like canines. Their diastema molars and premolars are flattened with ridges. Their teeth and upper jaw meet the lower jaw so that lateral movement of the lower jaw produces the grinding actions to break down plant materials. In herbivores, the incisors are dominant, the canines usually depressed, and the molars broad-topped.

As for the herbivore bowel, it usually runs almost 8 times longer than a carnivores (20 to 28 times the length of the body, from mouth to anus) since, unlike meat, plant matter is not prone to putrefaction, thus rendering quick elimination moot.

Herbivores also tend to have extended, compound stomachs.

Again, not much like us.

Omnivores (Roots, Berries, Meat, Whatever): Bears, Wild Pigs, Etc.

No animal is really adapted to eat all things; but if any animal comes close, it would have to be the bear. Typical foods consumed by bears include: ants, bees,

---

[1]Fast transit of waste for carnivores is important for two reasons. One, the faster the transit, the less opportunity for parasites to take hold. Two, meat tends to putrefy in the intestinal tract. Fast transit, therefore, limits exposure to the byproducts of putrefaction.

seeds, roots, nuts, berries, insect larvae such as grubs, and even flowers. Some meat, of course, is eaten by bears including rodents, fish, deer, pigs and lambs.[1] Grizzlies and Alaskan brown bears are well-known salmon eaters. And of course, anyone who has read *Winnie the Pooh* knows that many bears relish honey.

Other than the ants and grubs and rodents, the bear diet sounds a lot like the typical American diet; and, it's for this reason that many people conclude that the natural human diet is that of an omnivore. But remember, we're stepping back and taking a look physiologically where we fit in, and on those counts, we don't match the omnivores.

The biggest difference is in the teeth. Omnivores have the sharp canines of the carnivore **and** the pronounced incisors of the herbivore. They also have molars that are **both** pointed and broad-topped.

That's not even close to a human set of teeth.

Frugivores, Fruit and Nut Eaters: Gorillas, Etc.

In the frugivore, all the teeth are nearly of the same height. The canines are little projected and the molars are broad-topped. (Sound familiar?) Unlike the carnivore jaw, which as we have seen is vertically mobile for biting or tearing, the jaw of the typical frugivore is laterally mobile to allow for chewing.

As for the bowel of the frugivore, it runs about 10 to 12 times the length of the body from mouth to anus—the same as found in the human body.

The stomach of the frugivore is typically long and extended—a complex structure—containing $\frac{1}{10}$ of the acidic salts and pepsin found in a carnivore's stomach. Again, the same as in us.

So, here we have our match, but what does it mean? Are we restricted to fruits and nuts?

No, in fact, the frugivores we most closely resemble, the wild chimpanzees, periodically do indeed eat live insects and raw meat. Among the great apes (the gorilla,[2] the orangutan, the bonobo, and the chimpanzee) and ourselves, only humans and chimpanzees[3] hunt and eat meat on a frequent basis. But make no mistake, chimpanzees are largely fruit eaters, and meat comprises only about 3% of their diet—far, far less than is found in the typical American diet.

So Should We, or Should We Not, Eat Meat?

Is a vegetarian diet automatically better?

No, in fact, depending on blood type, some people actually do better when they include meat in their diet. Other factors in our diet affect our health to a much greater degree than whether or not we eat meat.

---

[1]Polar bears feed almost exclusively on seals and an occasional human; but then, what vegetation is there for them to eat in the frozen wastes of the Arctic.

[2]Gorillas have never been observed hunting or feeding on any animals other than invertebrates such as termites and ants.

[3]Wild chimps love fresh baby monkey meat.

So??

The bottom line is that eating small amounts of meat, chicken, or fish probably comes down mostly to a personal choice. If you choose to, you can eat 3 ounces a day, or less, of meat without any significant health problems—with the following provisos:

- Keep the amount small—3 ounces a day or less.
- Heavy consumption of meat significantly compromises beneficial bacteria in the colon resulting in a 1,000% increase in the levels of **harmful** bacteria in the colon and a concomitant 90% drop in the levels of the beneficial bacteria as measured in fecal matter.
- High consumption of meat also tends to push the body's pH levels into the acidic range, which as you'll see in Chapter 13 presents major health risks including cancer and osteoporosis.
- Epidemiological studies at Harvard Medical School showed that, "Men who eat red meat as a main dish five or more times a week have four times the risk of colon cancer than men who eat red meat less than once a month." They are also "more than twice as likely to get prostate cancer."
- If you're going to eat meat, buy only organic meat to avoid exposure to the whole range of chemicals,[1] growth hormones, and parasites present in beef and chicken, or the high levels of toxic metals present in most fish. If it isn't available locally, pressure your supermarket to carry it as an option.

2. What About Dairy?

The average American typically eats close to 600 pounds of dairy products a year, which makes it the single largest component of their diet. Unfortunately, this may not be as healthy as the milk ads you see on TV would lead you to believe. Even if the cow's milk you get is free of chemicals, growth hormones, allergenic proteins, blood, pus, antibiotics, bacteria, and viruses typically found in milk, you still have major problems. Cow's milk is not designed for people. For one thing, it has 20 times the casein of human milk.[2] (Human milk is designed to take an infant from 8 pounds to 40 pounds in 18 months. Cow's milk is designed to take a calf from 90 pounds to 1,000 pounds in about 24 months. Although they are both white, mother's milk and cow's milk

---

[1]Just as an example, over 90% of today's chickens are fed arsenic compounds. And while we're on the subject of chickens, it's probably worth mentioning that according to a government study, over 90% of the chickens sold in this country are infected with leukosis (chicken cancer). As for those chickens with too much cancerous tissue to be sold, well . . . they're destroyed, ground up, and fed back to the chickens that we ultimately buy and eat!!!

[2]The high levels of casein are just one of several reasons that humans do not digest milk proteins very well, leading to numerous allergic reactions and high levels of mucous in our noses and bowels. Incidentally, Elmer's® glue is made from cow's milk casein; that's why you see Elsie the cow on each bottle of Elmer's® glue.

are totally different beverages.) And for that matter, the cow's milk you buy in the store and the cow's milk that comes from a cow are not similar substances.

- First, homogenized milk is not natural and presents serious health risks. The theory behind homogenization sounds simple: break up the fat particles in milk until they are so small that they stay suspended in the milk and don't rise to the top and form the layer of cream that used to be the trademark of all bottles of milk. Unfortunately, there's a side effect to this process. Once you make the fat particles so small that they don't rise, you've also made them so small that they easily get absorbed into the body and clog your arteries.
- Second, there's the problem of the growth hormone used in dairy cows to increase milk production. This growth hormone, called bovine-somatotrophin[1] (BST), was developed by Monsanto. It was supposed to be identical to the actual growth hormone found in cows, and in fact, as part of their 55,000 page application to the FDA, Monsanto submitted a chart identifying the 191 amino acids contained in BST showing that they absolutely matched the amino acid chain found in natural growth hormone. Unfortunately, it seems, the application is inaccurate. The problem occurs at amino acid #144, which was supposed to be lysine in both the natural growth hormone and in Monsanto's BST. As it turns out, it isn't. In the July 1994, issue of *Protein Science* (3:1089-97, 1994), Bernard Violand, a Monsanto scientist published evidence that amino acid #144 in Monsanto's growth hormone is, in fact, epsilon-N-acetyllysine, a freak substance. Whoops! Ah, but then you probably think that once this problem came to light, totally nullifying the Monsanto application, that BST was recalled. Nope, not in the United States![2]

And then there's the fact that the body digests milk (any milk) differently once gastric juices begin to flow (at around 18–20 months old). Before gastric juices flow, milk is alkaline and non-mucous forming in the body; but once gastric juices enter the picture, they turn the milk acid, forming mucous, causing sinus problems, allergies, colds, etc. **That's why every animal except man weans its young off milk!** Think about that for a moment.

In addition to all of that, milk has been implicated in:

- Heart disease[3]

---

[1]Also called rBGH (recombinant bovine growth hormone).

[2]The FDA gave its approval for the sale of Monsanto's BST product back in 1993, but in Canada and the European Union, BST remains unapproved because of strong circumstantial evidence that it may promote cancer in cows and humans. Understand, this change in one amino acid is not insignificant. The replacement of one amino acid can change the configuration of a protein significantly; and configuration determines the properties and effects of a protein. Although the chemically detectable difference between true BGH and Monsanto's BST creation may be slight, the effects of the two hormones on the human body may be quite different indeed.

[3]If you do drink milk, it is essential that you take a folic acid supplement to neutralize the xanthine oxidase found in milk. Xanthine oxidase, which attacks the arteries, is a major factor in heart disease. Interestingly enough, this problem seems only to occur with homogenized milk. When nonhomogenized milk is consumed, the body excretes the xanthine oxidase.

- Cancer[1]—particularly breast cancer
- Diabetes[2]
- Allergies and colds
- Colitis
- Colic and earaches in young children

And finally, milk has played a major role in the development of the "super bacteria" that have recently emerged to plague our health. How? In 1990, the USDA allowed the dairy industry to increase the one part per hundred million antibiotic residue standard for milk by 10,000% to one part per million. The problem is that at this level of constant intake, the antibiotics actually destroy the probiotic colonies normally found in the intestinal tract, which then allows harmful bacteria to flourish and develop resistance to a whole range of antibiotics.[3]

If you must have dairy, use organic. Avoid homogenized milk at all costs. Also, there are a number of grain and rice-based milk alternatives, some of which are spectacular.

Note: milk is often pitched as a great source of calcium. It is not. Yes, it has a high calcium content, but the body is able to utilize very little of it; and, in fact, because of the way the body deals with milk, consumption of milk actually leaches calcium from the bones.[4] If you have any doubt about this, just consider the fact that **Americans are among the highest consumers of dairy in the world, eating an average of 600 pounds of dairy a year per person—and yet we have one of the highest incidences of osteoporosis in the civilized world!**

3. Unnatural Fats: The Number 1 Dietary Problem

Food manufacturers love hydrogenated oils because hydrogenation makes those oils thicker, creamier, and more appetizing to the consumer. Unfortunately, hydrogenation also saturates the oils' fatty acids, changing them into trans-fatty acids. Trans-fatty acids are the number one killer in our diets, and a major contributor to:

---

[1]It's worth noting that 60% of America's dairy cows are infected with the leukemia virus.

[2]One particular protein, beta-casein, found in cow's milk, can literally trick the immune system into attacking and destroying the insulin-producing beta cells of the pancreas.

[3]There are 52 different kinds of antibiotics and 59 bioactive hormones found in milk.

[4]It is a myth that we need milk for calcium. There are many far superior sources of calcium—such as sesame seeds. The problems with milk is that because of its high acidity, your body needs to buffer it with even more internal calcium than you get from the milk itself. Also, the 10 to 1 ratio of calcium to magnesium found in milk is insanely high and devastating to the body.

- Cancer
- Heart Disease
- Diabetes

Hydrogenated (and partially hydrogenated) oils are absolutely unnecessary and have no place in your diet or in any of the foods you eat. **The number one dietary prescription from this chapter is to totally eliminate all hydrogenated oils from your diet.** Unfortunately, it's not as easy as it sounds. Food manufacturers have put them in almost every food they manufacture. The good news is that if enough people refuse to buy foods that contain trans-fatty acid oils, manufacturers will stop putting them in their foods.

You also want to eliminate refined oils and manufactured polyunsaturated oils from your diet. What oils are good? Virtually any raw natural oil is good. Olive oil is the best. Use lots of extra virgin olive oil in your cooking. Surprisingly, butter is cool—provided that you can get butter that doesn't contain antibiotics and bovine growth hormone and all the rest of the nonsense that many dairy farmers use.

"Wait a second! Isn't butter high in saturated fat?" Absolutely, and let's put that bugaboo to rest. Natural saturated fats in moderation are not a problem. They do not raise cholesterol levels. They do not lead to heart disease. In fact, there is actually a diet that helps people lose weight, and lower cholesterol levels while eating as much meat and eggs and natural saturated fat as they like.[1] The two reasons this diet works are (1) natural saturated fats do not cause heart problems, and (2) all versions of this diet call for the elimination of snack foods, processed foods, sugared foods, foods containing any trans-fatty acids, and foods high on the glycemic index.

4. Refined Carbohydrates: The Number 2 Dietary Problem

This includes all refined and processed foods, including:

- Everything made with white flour
- White rice
- Cold cereals
- Most hot cereals
- Most snack foods

---

[1] I've already discussed my concerns with too much meat in the diet; nevertheless, these programs do demonstrate the health-building power of just eliminating the bad things from our diet.

- All sugar foods, including cakes, candies, and soda pop[1]

They negatively affect the body in a number of ways. They are all acid forming in the body, which we'll talk more about in Chapter 13. They are all converted to triglycerides in the body and stored as fat. And they all rank high on the glycemic index (with no redeeming nutritional value such as the fruits and vegetables that are also high on the glycemic index).

THE GLYCEMIC INDEX

The glycemic index, and identifying high-glycemic foods, is one of the hot areas of nutritional science right now. Not to make light of it, it is an extremely important dietary consideration, but with one huge **however.** First, though, a quick discussion of the glycemic index.

Diabetics have been using the glycemic index for years to help in controlling their insulin levels. Quite simply, foods that adversely affect blood sugar by elevating insulin levels are termed "high glycemic" foods, and foods that do not elevate insulin levels are "low glycemic." High glycemic foods can:

- Cause your body to store fat
- Make you fatigued
- Cause your brain to go "fuzzy"
- Lead to heart problems such as elevated LDL cholesterol levels and high blood pressure

Obviously, these are conditions to be avoided. High glycemic foods that cause elevated insulin levels and the concomitant problems I just mentioned include:

- Bananas
- Raisins
- Carrots
- Potatoes
- Corn
- Breads, cereals, pastas, and rice of all kinds

---

[1]Soda pop, particularly colas, may be the single worst "food" ever invented. First, soda contains approximately 1 teaspoon of sugar per ounce of soda. (Aspartame is even worse—once having been considered by the military for possible use as a battlefield neurotoxin.) That works out to about 12 teaspoons per can, or 32 teaspoons per Big Gulp. Many sodas, particularly colas, are high in phosphoric acid, which leaches calcium out of your body at an astounding rate. And all sodas "feature" CO_2 bubbles, which when you think about it, is the body's main waste product!

- Virtually all snack foods
- Sugars of all kinds and soda pop

Earlier, I mentioned that there was a big **however** to the glycemic index. What is that however? It's called chewing. If you chew your food well enough, the saliva neutralizes almost all of the glycemic response. So how much do you need to chew your food?

There's an old saying that says, "You should drink your solids and chew your liquids." What that means is that you should chew the dry food you eat until it turns to liquid in your mouth (about 40 chews per mouthful), and that you should swish liquids back and forth in your mouth (chew them as it were) an equal number of times.

As we've already discussed when we talked about refined foods, you should give up snack foods and refined flour products and sugar sweetened foods for a number of reasons. On the other hand, for most people, if you chew them enough, it's still okay to eat all of the fresh fruits and vegetables you want—even if they are high on the glycemic index.

General Recommendations

- Diet. Clean up your act.
  - Eliminate as much of the processed and cooked food from your diet as possible. Instead of canned or frozen, eat fresh.
  - Eliminate as much of the refined flours, grains, and sugars as possible. Instead of white bread, eat **real** whole wheat. Instead of cake and ice cream for dessert, eat fruit.
  - Replace low-value foods such as potatoes and iceberg lettuce with high value foods such as sweet potatoes and almost any of the richly colored vegetables (particularly, spinach, brussels sprouts, broccoli, and beets).[1]
  - As much as possible, eliminate all snack foods and fast foods. Replace with prunes (no kidding, an extremely powerful antioxidant), raisins, and all of the berries.
  - Eliminate **all** hydrogenated oils and trans-fatty acids. Replace with olive oil and fresh butter.
  - Cut back on the quantity of meat, pork,[2] chicken, and dairy in your diet.

---

[1]For those with arthritis, it might be useful to forego vegetables from the nightshade family, including tomatoes, spinach, and eggplant.

[2]And no, pork is not "the other white meat." In fact, pork is probably one of the more indigestible meats you can eat.

And make sure that what you do consume is organic.[1] Fish, of course, is okay—okay that is, if you can be sure it's free of heavy metals and toxins and hormonal "modifications."

- So what does that leave you? Actually thousands of choices. Virtually, everything that we've talked about eliminating is easily replaced with a healthier version. **If you can't find the organic meats and dairy you want, or the whole grain foods you're looking for, talk to your supermarket. In most cases, they will get it if you ask.**
- Of course, if someone is in an advanced state of illness, they better clean up their act totally, and eat no meat and no cooked food. In fact, ideally, they should go on a raw juice fast[2]—at least, until they get well. Once you're well, you can bake up a potato, or grill yourself a nice piece of organic beef (if that's your bent).
- **The bottom line is that the worse you eat, the more often you will need to cleanse and detox and make use of supplements.**

So After All That, What Do I Eat?

At one time, I was totally vegetarian, primarily for ethical reasons. Anyone who has any awareness of how cattle, poultry, and pigs are treated in our modern "superfarms," must think twice about consuming products produced by this system. It is incredibly cruel.

Unfortunately, after years of speaking engagements in numerous places around the world, I got tired of eating iceberg lettuce with second-rate Italian dressing for lunch, and white rice and dead vegetables for dinner. I broke down and started eating small amounts of chicken and fish.

My diet now consists of:

- Fresh juices, superfoods, and ground flaxseed (see next chapter) for breakfast.
- Large fresh salads with a variety of greens and vegetables[3] with the occasional small piece of chicken or fish for lunch.

---

[1]Incidentally, pesticide levels are far more concentrated in the animal flesh and dairy we eat than in the fruits and vegetables sprayed with these pesticides. Think about it for a moment. The animals consume these pesticides day after day, steadily concentrating all of the pesticides they eat through their entire lives in their flesh. The bottom line is that the higher up the food chain you go, the more concentrated the pesticides are. A cow eats hundreds of pounds of clover to make a few gallons of milk—concentrating the pesticide in that milk. Then again, it takes 21 pounds of milk to make 1 pound of butter, and 10 pounds of milk to make 1 pound of cheese—concentrating the pesticides even more.

[2]See Chapter 13.

[3]Sometimes I'll substitute a plate of lightly steamed or baked vegetables for the salad.

- Dinner is light. Sometimes a bowl of slow cooked whole-grain cereal so the enzymes are still active. Sometimes a small bowl of soup. Sometimes fresh fruit, etc.

- On the other hand, I still have an occasional slice of pizza. When I was young, I'd eat pizza 2–3 times a week. Now it's once a month. And more often than I should, I still indulge a sweet tooth and have dessert.

CHAPTER 7

VITAMINS, MINERALS, AND PHYTOCHEMICALS

WHY WE NEED TO SUPPLEMENT

You often hear doctors say that there's no need to supplement if you eat a balanced diet. If only that were true. Unfortunately, the food we eat today is not the same as the food we ate 50–100 years ago. We have to compensate for the loss of "value" in our food.

- It takes 80 cups of today's supermarket spinach to give you the same iron you'd get from just one cup of spinach grown 50 years ago.
- According to a Rutgers University study, it now takes 19 ears of corn to equal the nutritional value of just one ear of corn grown in 1940.
- There is less than half the protein in today's wheat as in the wheat our grandparents ate.
- Much of our soil is so depleted that our farm crops depend **entirely** on the chemical fertilizers they are fed to grow. That means that most of the food we eat is devoid of virtually all the trace minerals we need for survival.
- And on and on.

When you think about it, it doesn't take a rocket scientist to figure out what's happened. We've exchanged quality for quantity. You can't keep increasing your yield per acre, at the same time steadily depleting your soil year after year, and not expect to lose something in the process. And what's been lost is the quality of our food.

Organic vs Non-Organic

As we've just seen, most of the food sold in our supermarkets is nutritionally compromised. Part of the solution lies in organic foods, which hearken back to the more nutritionally beneficial foods of 50 years ago. Consider the following comparisons between organic and conventionally grown food.

- Organic snap beans have 30 times the manganese, 22 times the iron, and 23 times the copper of the conventionally grown variety.
- Organic cabbage has four times the calcium and four times the potassium of the cabbage you buy in the supermarket.
- Organic lettuce is five times higher in calcium, 50 times higher in iron, and 170 times higher in manganese.
- Organic tomatoes are 12 times higher in magnesium, 68 times higher in manganese, and almost 2,000 times higher in iron.

And then there's the difference between organic and **super organic.** Super organic, when you can find it, has on average, **twice** the nutritional value of standard organic (which, as we've already seen, has several times the food value of conventionally grown food). To give you a sense of the extent of these differences, consider:

- Conventional farms use no compost at all in the growing of their crops. Instead, they rely on chemical fertilizers that have a limited range of nutrients—just what the plant requires to grow, which is why they are so deficient in the nutrients that people need. (And of course, we won't even talk about taste.)
- The average organic farm uses about 3–5 tons of organic matter/compost per acre per year.
- The average super organic farm will use upwards of 100 tons of organic matter per acre per year.

Nutritional Stress

A second factor we have to consider is nutritional stress. We're just exposed to far more environmental and pollution stresses than our bodies were ever designed to handle—more than the human body has ever before been required to handle in the history of the world. Even if you were able to consume an all-organic, optimized diet, it takes far more of the protective phytochemicals that food provides than we can possibly get in our diets—even if the food we ate was of the highest quality. Our bodies were never designed to handle:

- High levels of radiation from dental x-rays and high-altitude airplane flights
- Organo-phosphate nerve-gas pesticide residues
- Totally artificial fats (hydrogenated oils, trans-fatty acids, and homogenized fat)
- High levels of refined sugar (with the average American now consuming over 137 pounds a year)

- A totally fiberless white flour diet (including, breads, pastas, cakes, pop tarts, pastries, tortillas, etc.)
- Constant exposure to disruptive electromagnetic fields
- Chlorines and fluorides in our water
- Continued, unrelenting, high-stress jobs and living situations

The bottom line is that if you live in any industrialized country in the world today, you must supplement to maintain your health—to reduce the risk of cancer, heart disease, degenerative diseases of all kinds, retard the aging process, and protect against toxic injury.

And What Do We Supplement With?

Before we can actually determine which supplements we need to take, we need to take a quick look at the fundamentals of nutrition.

Proteins, Fats, and Carbohydrates

For many people, this is where their nutritional knowledge begins and ends. They count calories and compare ratios of fat calories to total calories. In most hospitals, the sole concern of the certified nutritionists who prepare hospital "food" is putting together a proper balance of proteins, fats, and carbohydrates. As you will soon learn, this is tantamount to nutritional insanity.

- Proteins are essential for the growth and repair of all body tissue. Proteins are made of amino acids, some of which your body can produce by itself, and some of which must be included in your diet.
  - A great deal is made about the need for protein, but the fact is our protein requirements are not really very large and are easy to fill. To figure out your protein requirement, just divide your weight in half. That's your daily protein requirement in grams. If you want to rough that out in ounces, it works out to about 30 grams per ounce. In other words, if you weigh 150 pounds, you need 75 grams (2½ ounces) of protein a day.
  - Theoretically, milk is a top-rated protein, but in reality it's not. As we've already discussed, it messes up the pH which results in incomplete digestion. Meat and fish are fine. Eggs are too. Surprisingly, though, some of the best sources are actually vegetarian. Spirulina and chlorella are both not only higher in actual percentage of protein (60–80% vs 20–25% for animal sources) but also in terms of bioavailablity.
- Fats are the ultimate energy storage system. Your body stores fat for long-term energy use. Think of bears who live off their fat for months at a time while they hibernate. On the other hand, if you're eating every day, your

body doesn't really need to store fat for future use. Nevertheless, certain fats are essential for life and health.

- •• Essential Fatty Acids, or EFA's, are among the approximately 50–70 nutrients that have been "identified" as necessary to sustain human life and good health. Unlike saturated fats, EFA's remain liquid at body temperature and, because of their bent shape, they do not dissolve into each other and clog our arteries.
- •• In point of fact, all fats are actually fatty acids, consisting of one part fat (which is not water soluble) and one part acid (which is). What makes Omega-3 (the king of EFA's), Omega-6, and Omega-9 so important is that not only are they good for you—they are, in fact, essential. And what's more, your body can't produce them, which means you must get them in your diet. However, **due to the extreme sensitivity of EFA's to light and oxygen, they have been removed from virtually all processed foods so that the foods have a longer shelf life.**
- •• The sad fact is that our lack of EFA's has been linked to many of today's diseases and afflictions including hair loss, lack of energy, skin problems, heart and circulatory problems, and all of the immune disorders (including arthritis).
- •• **The reason EFA's are so important is that they are the main components of all cellular membranes—inside and out—where they protect against viruses, bacteria, and allergens.** They are the key building blocks of all fats and oils, both in our foods and in our bodies. They play a key role in the construction and maintenance of nerve cells and the hormone-like substances called prostaglandins and help decrease cholesterol and triglyceride levels in the blood.
- •• **The bottom line is that essential fatty acids are vital to our health. They quite literally are the primary healing agents in the body, and according to some estimates, as many as 90% of all people are deficient in at least one of them.**

- Carbohydrates are the body's short-term energy foods. Simple carbohydrates, such as sugar and white flour are utilized by the body in a matter of minutes. Complex carbohydrates take time to break down and are, therefore, utilized over a matter of hours.
  - •• The best carbohydrates are fresh fruits and vegetables—pure and simple. Buy organic. Wash thoroughly.

Minerals

Your body is actually made mostly of minerals and water. As it turns out, your overall health is determined far more by minerals than proteins, fats, carbohydrates, or even vitamins. Calcium, for example, is not only used to build strong bones and teeth, but is present in **every single cell in the body** and is instrumental in the transporting of nutrients in and out of those cells.

- Want some iron? Why not grind down a nail and eat the shavings. Want some calcium? Why not do what the Three Stooges do and shuck some oysters, throw the meat away, and eat the shells. Sound silly? Well what do you think is in most of the vitamin pills you buy?
- Well then, how about this as an alternative? Want some iron? How about eating some beets. Want some calcium? How about ground sesame seeds or collard greens or carrot juice?
- The bottom line is that your body can't handle straight minerals. They carry an electric charge which is opposite that of your intestinal wall so that they stick to the wall and can't pass through. Once stuck to the intestinal wall, they are "pushed" along and out of the body. In the end, you absorb only about 3–5% of the straight minerals you consume. Many supplement makers use chelation to mask the electric charge (thereby tricking your body into absorbing the minerals).
- On the other hand, plants pull minerals straight out of the ground, and then biologically transform them into the very substance of the plant itself. Not surprisingly, your body likes this form of mineral better.

Trace Minerals

For years, trace minerals were virtually ignored when it came to nutrition. In fact, in the early days of vitamin/mineral supplements, it was rare to even find them included. Since then, however, primarily due to discoveries made in the large-scale raising of cattle, hogs, and chickens, we have learned that trace minerals are among the most important components of good health—and even life itself.

A full complement of the 72–84 trace elements is essential for optimum health.

Vitamins

The dictionary defines a vitamin as "an organic compound naturally occurring in plant and animal tissue and that is essential in small amounts for the control of metabolic processes." A more illuminating definition is that vitamins are coenzymes. Their primary role is to help your body's enzymes do their job.[1] When vitamins are available in limited amounts, enzyme reactions are inhibited.

---

[1]For example, the enzyme responsible for breaking down alcohol, alcohol dehydrogenase, uses vitamin B6 (pyridoxine) as its cofactor.

Phytochemicals

Phytochemicals are the hot "new" discoveries in nutritional science. They include things such as sulforaphane from broccoli, resveratrol from grapes, and lycopene from tomatoes. Another way of looking at phytochemicals is simply as vitamins and antioxidants in the process of being discovered. This is not necessarily a quick process. It took 50 years for Vitamin E to be declared a vitamin after it was discovered.

It's Not That Simple

You would think that supplementation would be pretty easy. Figure out just where people are likely to be deficient, then make a pill that supplements for those suspected deficiencies—sort of a one-a-day multiple-vitamin kind of thing. Determining the best supplement to take would then be a simple job of reading the label.

Unfortunately, it's not that simple. There are actually several problems.

1. Natural and synthetic vitamins are not necessarily the same thing.
2. In nature, nutrients do not exist in isolation; they exist in *nutrient complexes.* And as it turns out, our bodies require the complexes, not the isolates.

Natural vs Synthetic

Actually, vitamins can be classified as either totally natural, co-natural, or synthetic.

Totally Natural

Almost no vitamins that you buy are totally natural. Why? Quite simply, cost. Direct extraction of vitamins from foods is prohibitively expensive. For example, acerola cherries, the best natural source of vitamin C, contain only 1 percent of vitamin C by weight. Most supplements that list acerola cherries as their vitamin C source contain only a small percentage of vitamin C from the cherries—the rest is synthesized vitamin C.

Co-natural

Co-natural vitamins are derived from vegetable and animal sources through the use of solvent extraction, distillation, hydrolysis, or crystallization—**but, by definition, haven't undergone any conversion or chemical alteration during the extraction process.**

Synthetic

Synthetic vitamins can be derived from either natural or chemical sources. **What makes them synthetic is that they undergo a process of "conversion," either as a result of the extraction process or as the result of pure chemical buildup.**[1] Synthetics are, at best, about 50% as effective as natural vitamins and may actually suppress the body's ability to absorb the natural portion of the vitamin.

What You Actually Get in the Store

Many commercial-grade vitamin and mineral concentrates are synthesized by the large pharmaceutical and chemical companies[2] from the same starting material that they make their drugs from (coal tar, wood pulp, petroleum products, animal byproducts, waste and fecal matter, ground rocks, stones, shells, and metal.)

- Most Vitamin B-12 (cobalamine) is made from activated sewage sludge—and then stabilized with cyanide (thus becoming, cyanocobalamine)
- Most vitamin D is made from irradiated oil
- The bulk of all vitamin E is produced in the labs at Kodak
- Niacinamide is made by boiling sulfur in the presence of asbestos
- Supplemental calcium, for the most part, is either mined from the earth, ground from old bones, or made by grinding up oyster shells

Another surprise is that the term organic, when applied to supplements, does not mean the same thing as it does with food. For supplements, all the word organic means is that the molecule contains at least one carbon atom (as in organic chemistry). **In other words, a supplement can be labeled 100% organic and not be natural at all.**

Many so-called natural vitamins have synthetics added to "increase potency," or to standardize the amount in a capsule or batch. Many vitamins also add a synthetic salt form of the vitamin to increase stability. These synthetics are easily identified by the terms acetate, bitartrate, chloride, gluconate, hydrochloride, nitrate, and succinate.

---

[1]Light passing through a natural vitamin always bends to the right due to its molecular rotation. Synthetic vitamins behave differently. That same ray of light splits into two parts when passing through a synthetic–one part bending to the right (d for dexorotary), the other to the left (l for levorotary). A natural vitamin E fraction, for example, is easily identified by the "d-alpha tocopherol." the synthetic by "dl-alpha-tocopherol." (Incidentally, the body can't use the l-form of vitamin E, and the l-form may even inhibit the d-form from entering cell membranes.)

[2]Kodak, Hoffman La Roche, etc.

The Bigger Problem

Modern medicine refuses to define the human body as a holistic entity, but rather as a grouping of separate parts and pieces. Not surprisingly, that same paradigm has been applied to nutrition. In other words, modern nutrition is based on the concept that key nutrients can be identified and isolated. Unfortunately, the reality is quite different.

- Fifteen years ago, vitamin C (ascorbic acid) was all the rage. Then, suddenly, after years of people scarfing down ascorbic acid, it was discovered that your body really couldn't absorb ascorbic acid very well unless the bioflavonoids, hesperidin, and rutin were present. So, suddenly, all vitamin C was sold **with** the bioflavonoids, hesperidin, and rutin. Then it was discovered that you really couldn't absorb vitamin C very well (even if the bioflavonoids, hesperidin, and rutin were present) unless calcium was also present. So again, suddenly, all vitamin C was sold **with** calcium. Two questions that any thoughtful person might want to ask are:
    - What value were people getting all those years they were consuming just ascorbic acid?
    - Was there any source for vitamin C available for all those years that packed ascorbic acid with its bioflavonoids and calcium? And the answer is: of course! Oranges package the whole deal together. Grapefruits package the whole deal together. Acerola cherries package the whole deal together. Nature packages the whole deal together!
- Several years ago, Beta Carotene was "discovered." Suddenly, Beta Carotene supplements were everywhere. At first the press was touting the anti-cancer properties of Beta Carotene. Then they were touting other studies that proved that it didn't prevent cancer.[1] Then, forget Beta Carotene; suddenly, everyone was touting another carotenoid, lycopene. Lycopene prevents prostate cancer. Then there was Lutein, also a carotenoid. Lutein prevents macular degeneration. But once again, if we turn to nature, we see that nature already packed all of these things together in a complex. The seaweed, Dunaliella salina, for example, contains all of the popular carotenoids plus a whole slew of others, such as Alpha carotene and Zeaxanthin. Carrots, for that matter, contain approximately 400 different carotenoids in addition to Beta Carotene, and many of those carotenoids are far more powerful than Beta Carotene.
- A third example is the mineral chromium. Over the past few years, the synthetic versions of chromium, chromium picolinate and chromium polynicotinate, have been all the rage. They're even promoted as being "better" than

---

[1] Both negative studies evaluated a synthetic Beta Carotene. For what it's worth, almost all of the Beta Carotene on the market today is an isolated synthetic made from acetylene gas. Yummy!

the original, but as it turns out, that's not entirely true. In its natural state, chromium comes packed with a whole complex of substances called GTF (glucose tolerance factor), which, among other things, protects against diabetes. Chromium picolinate and chromium polynicotinate, because they are isolates, do not contain GTF.

I could go on and on giving examples, such as the B vitamins and vitamin E, where science has continually come up short in identifying the key factors that make it all work. The bottom line, though, is that in nature, vitamins do not exist in isolation; they exist in complexes.

And here's a final thought for you. Although it is conceivable that science may someday identify all of the key nutrients contained in nature so that we don't keep finding out what nutrients we forgot to include, it is an impossibility that science will ever identify how all of these nutrients interact with and support each other. The mathematical possibilities are just too immense. In the end, we will find that there are literally thousands of nutrients that our bodies require to remain healthy,[1] and the possibilities for the synergistic interaction of all of these nutrients is astronomical.

How Much to Take for Each

In the early 1940s a program was established to determine the Minimum Daily Requirement (MDR) you would need of each essential nutrient to prevent the onset of disease. Testing was simple. Withhold a certain nutrient (let's say vitamin C) until disease (in this case, scurvy) appeared. At that point, the appropriate nutrient was introduced back into the diet until the disease disappeared. The amount that it took to make the disease go away was the MDR. The RDA (Recommended Daily Allowance) was then established as a small percentage (to allow a safety margin) above the MDR. Recently, RDA was replaced by the term DV (Daily Value), and even more recently by the term RDI (Recommended Dietary Intake).

The problem with this whole approach is that it deals only with short-term deficiencies. What are the long term implications (10, 20, 30 years down the line) of nutritional deficiency? The answer is now becoming apparent for all but the blind to see: an epidemic of cancer, heart disease, diabetes, osteoporosis, etc. **And what makes it all even more ludicrous, is that as pathetically low as the RDA/DV/RDI is, a USDA government survey of 21,500 people found that *not one single person* consumed 100% of the US. RDA, from the foods they ate.**

---

[1]As I've already mentioned, there are some 400 carotenoids that have been identified. Each day there are new phytochemicals, not to mention whole new classes of phytochemicals, being identified. And new antioxidants are being identified, almost daily it seems.

General Recommendations

Overall Supplement

So the question remains, what's the best overall (one-a-day kind of thing) supplement? The best way to look at the question of an overall supplement is to break it into three categories: Optimum, Acceptable, and Avoid At All Costs.

Optimum

- One good choice is to use concentrated "food-based" vitamin complexes. Such supplements will contain concentrated forms of liver, yeast, and wheat germ for example.
- Another good choice is to use "food-grown" supplements. Instead of being chemically manufactured, food-grown supplements are cultivated using a live biodynamic growing process. Literally, by growing nutritional yeast in a "super-dense nutrient-broth," you end up with a "living" vitamin/mineral complex that is comprised of a highly complex interlocking system of vitamins, enzymes, minerals, active bioflavonoid groups, microproteins, complex carbohydrates, and countless other naturally occurring food constituents.
- A third alternative is a superfood combination that contains things like rice bran, spirulina, chlorella, flower pollen, nutritional yeast, wheat grass, barley grass, powdered beets, etc. to provide a full complement of vitamins and minerals.
  - Watch out for fillers. Superfoods are expensive, and many manufacturers cheat their formulas down by adding large amounts of things such as low-grade rice bran and lecithin.[1] Also, it's important to make sure that your superfood provides good sources for the B vitamins and for vitamin D.
  - For many years, it was thought that edible seaweeds, fermented soya foods, and spirulina contained high levels of B12. They don't. What they contain are B12 analogues (chemical lookalikes) which your body cannot use. You'll need another source of B12.
  - Recent studies have found that more than half of all people have too little vitamin D in their bodies. The big surprise was that ⅓ of those who were deficient were taking vitamin D supplements. Make sure your superfood provides adequate amounts of vitamin D—and get some sunlight on your body.

---

[1]Don't get me wrong. These are not bad things; they're just not nutrient dense. Their primary value is that they're relatively inexpensive.

Acceptable

- It's possible to find high-quality vitamin/mineral supplements at the health food store that use only co-natural vitamins and no synthetics. The problem with supplements **based** on co-naturals is that they can never be complete. What co-naturals are great for is "spiking up" a supplement based on one of our Optimum options. An example would be a "food-based" supplement augmented with co-natural vitamins E and C.

Avoid At All Costs

- Supplements made from synthetics are not an option. At their best, they are only 50% as effective as a natural vitamin. At their worst, they actually may carry harmful side effects.

Essential Fatty Acids

Since EFA's have been removed from virtually all of the foods we normally eat, supplementation is essential. The best sources for EFA's are:

- If you're taking your daily dose of ground flaxseed as recommended in Chapter 3, you will be getting all of the alpha-linolenic acid you need. Otherwise, you will want to supplement with 1–2 tablespoons daily of organic, cold-pressed, high-lignan flaxseed oil.
- Borage oil is more potent and less expensive than evening primrose or black current oil and is the best choice for gamma linolenic acid.
- Fish oil provides DHA (docosahexaenoic acid) and EPA (eicosapentaenoic acid).
- Recently a variation of a long-chain fatty acid cetyl ester called Omega-9 Plus™ has been discovered. Although not yet officially designated an Essential Fatty Acid, supplementation with this fatty acid has shown a remarkable ability to relieve pain, reverse the effects of arthritis, and relieve the symptoms of a whole host of diseases.

Trace Minerals

There are now many good sources of trace minerals available. You will see them described as "colloidal minerals" or "ionic minerals" or "sea minerals." Take your pick and use one. Trace mineral deficiency is epidemic in America because of the poor quality of our diets. Supplementation is essential.

Phytonutrients

At the moment, the best source is still real food. Foods you will want to include in your diet include things such as:

- Soy products of all kinds for the genistein and the isoflavones
- Broccoli, brussel sprouts, and kale for the sulforaphane
- Garlic and onions for the allyl sulfides
- Red grapes (including seeds) for the proanthocyanidins and the resveratrol
- Green tea for the polyphenols

CHAPTER 8

MIRACLE HERBS

Right now, herbs are "hot." Major companies are going herbal. The AMA is acknowledging the value of some herbs. Herbs are being featured in the cover stories of major magazines such as *Time* and *Newsweek.* Sales of herbs are well into the billions of dollars a year. This is a time for herbalists and alternative healers to celebrate. Right?

Not necessarily.

While many in the alternative health community have fought for recognition from the medical establishment, personally, I have been very wary of it. And now that recognition has come, I believe we are about to pay the price.

What specifically is the problem? The answer lies in one word: "co-option" (definition: to take over an independent minority movement through assimilation into an established group or culture).

STANDARDIZATION

Almost everyone now believes that standardized extracts are a good thing. They answer the medical community's need for predictable doses and effects. All of the top herbal manufacturers now promote their use of standardized herbs. To a large degree, though I believe it's a red herring. I'm not a big fan of standardization. Let me explain.

To understand what standardization means, let's take a look at orange juice. The orange juice you buy in the store, either in half gallon containers or frozen concentrate, is actually a great example of a standardized herbal product (oranges fitting in the broad definition of herbs).[1] The manufacturers of these juice products have been able to identify the "active ingredients" of orange juice that are primarily responsible for taste. In the case of orange juice, those key ingredients are sugar (sweetness) and acid (tartness). Now the way standardization works with orange juice is that if a manufacturer finds that a batch of oranges is not sweet enough, they'll blend that batch with a much sweeter batch to bring it up to the "ideal" sweetness. If that same batch is too acidic, they'll blend it with a batch that's less acidic, until their testing shows it's reached just

---

[1]An herb being defined as "any of various often aromatic plants used especially in medicine or as seasoning."

the right level of acidity. That's why each can or container of orange juice you buy tastes pretty much like the one you bought the week before. That's standardization. So what's my problem?

Have you ever tasted a can of frozen orange juice or juice from a container that even comes close to the taste of good fresh squeezed?[1] That's the problem. While standardization can make one batch virtually identical to the next, it can never make any batch as good as really good non-standardized fresh squeezed. Why?

The reason is simple. The taste of orange juice is governed by far more factors than sugar and acid. It is the result of the interplay of dozens and dozens of natural flavors, esters, and oils which are beyond the ability of any manufacturer to control. It is a symphony of taste—a symphony that we cannot duplicate by tweaking one or two "active" ingredients. (And, in fact, tweaking is actually often deleterious in the sense that it destroys the "natural" balance of all those flavors and esters that are not standardized.)

Let's consider another example: wine. Has anyone ever been able to guarantee in a laboratory the taste of the best wines? Of course not. The taste of the wine is the result of the soil the grapes are grown in and the temperature and rains that occur in a given year. Now here comes an important point. While it's true that the quality of wine at any vineyard may vary from year to year, is it not also true that the best vineyards consistently produce the best wines? Some years, a great vineyard may produce superb wine. The next year, the wine may only be outstanding or really good. But isn't it true that a great vineyard will almost **always** produce a better tasting wine than Ripple—a standardized wine, if you will?

And that's the problem with standardization. It lowers the bar of what we can expect from herbal formulations. Standardized formulas will never match the quality (and healing power) of a non-standardized formula **made from the highest quality herbs** because the standardized formula seeks to control one, two or three "identified" active ingredients at the expense of all the other "active" ingredients that we don't yet know about. **Standardization "distorts" plant synergy, and it disrupts the natural ratios of active ingredients inherent in the plant itself and replaces them with "arbitrary" ratios as determined by today's researchers.**

And then, of course, in addition to everything else, our attempt to identify active ingredients is fundamentally flawed. The procedure used is right out of standard drug testing: isolate individual chemical components and test their effects—one at a time. If a particular biochemical from an herb tests as "non-active," we can eliminate it from standardization of that herb. But what if that component has a different value in the grand scheme of things? What if, although it may do nothing by itself, its presence makes another component twice as effective? What if....

---

[1]Keeping in mind that there are people who actually prefer the taste of Sunny Delight.

An obvious question has to be occurring to you right now: "If what I'm saying is true, then why is 'everybody' standardizing their herbs now?" And the answer is that standardization is the herbalist's answer to traditional medicine's complaint that herbs are unpredictable. Another way of saying this, which may be more illuminating, is that standardized extracts make herbs more like drugs. But as we've just seen, herbs are not like drugs. Herbs are not single chemicals. They are a synergistic blend of natural compounds. Once you acknowledge this, the whole idea of standardization is revealed for what it is: co-option.

So what's the alternative? Well, one thing that we do know about herbs, through centuries of use, is that high-quality herbs have great healing powers. We also know that well-grown herbs are consistently high in all active ingredients—those that we can identify, and those that we won't know about for another hundred years. The bottom line, then, is that if you must guarantee something, then why not:

- Use high-quality herbs with their natural ratios of ingredients. This means, of course, that you can't "doctor up" poor-quality herbs as you can with standardization.
- Guarantee a **minimum** level for all active ingredients (as we know them today).
- This alternative provides all of the advantages of standardization, and none of the negatives.

An Interesting Development

Several companies are taking standardization to the next level by running herbs through the same lab tests that prescription medicines must pass—called bioassays—to uncover just what biologically active ingredients they contain. Using certain test-tube experiments, for example, they can test whether a chemical interacts with the brain pathways involved in depression. If the experiments measure a response, that chemical is biologically active. Already, these companies claim that their new testing process has discovered that there are some five active ingredients that may help St. John's Wort ease depression—not the single ingredient, hypericin, which is currently the target of standardization.

These companies are also looking to contract with herb manufacturers to "guarantee" their herbal products. American Home Products, for example, has already begun marketing six PharmaPrint-tested herbs under its popular Centrum supplement brand.

And finally, these same companies also plan to seek **FDA approval to sell the most effective herbs as prescription drugs.** This will allow doctors to sell, for a higher price of course, a "fully tested medicine version" of the same herbs you currently buy in the health store.

There are four fundamental problems I see with this whole process:

1. First, as we've already alluded to, no testing process in the world can test for the synergistic factor of all the biochemical components in herbs. No testing process can determine if a compound, even though it may not be biologically active itself, serves to increase the biological activity of another compound. That's why no testing process can match the skill of the professional herbalist (just as it cannot come close to matching the palate of the professional wine taster) in determining the effectiveness of an herb.

2. It reinforces the paradigm of herbs as drugs (that is, for symptom X, take herb Y) and puts herbal medicine in the hands of doctors (who, as a rule, have no understanding of herbal medicine) and takes it out of the hands of the herbal professionals.

3. It actually leads to the classification of herbs as drugs, as both companies are already looking to do.

4. It totally ignores the other aspects of herbal quality.

Interestingly enough, this is not a new idea. We've gone down this road before—with disastrous consequences. The modern drug industry, as we know it today, was created out of herbal medicine. (The word "drug" itself actually comes from the old German word "droge," which was used to describe the process of "drying" herbs in preparation for use.) The apparent motive behind the development of pharmaceuticals was to create purer, more potent, and more effective "medicines." Unfortunately, as we now know, the net result was, in many cases, just the opposite—less effective medicines with a whole range of deadly side effects. Pharmaceuticals, however, do offer one major advantage over herbs. They are patentable, and as such, generate billions and billions of dollars in profits for the companies that manufacture them—and the medical system that distributes them.

Herb Quality

Ninety-nine percent of the herbs used by American companies do not come from the US. They are imported from Eastern Europe and from many third-world countries such as India, China, and Mexico.

Unfortunately, these countries use large amounts of insecticides and pesticides in the growing of their herbs. DDT is still commonly used in Asia and Mexico, whereas organo-phosphate nerve-gas based insecticides are commonly used throughout Eastern Europe.

It's also worth noting that most of the areas in which these herbs are grown in these countries are heavily polluted. The herbs are inundated by polluted rain and irrigated by polluted rivers. In Eastern Europe, for example, there have been no environmental laws for decades. Rivers have been used as open sewers. Everything from chemical toxic waste to radioactive waste—no joke—has been dumped into these rivers.

The reason most American companies use these herb sources, regardless of the problems just mentioned, is that they are cheap. Good quality organic and wildcrafted herbs cost as much as 20 times more. Before you use any company's herbal formulations, you should learn where their herbs come from.

Herbal Preparation

There are a number of ways herbs can be prepared. In increasing order of potency, they are:

1. Fresh herb
2. Dried herbs are more concentrated because the water has been removed. Dried herbs can be ground up and put in pills, or capsules
3. Teas
4. Commercial[1] tinctures
5. Commercial liquid concentrate (like a tincture, but with some of the fluid removed)
6. Commercial dried concentrate (no liquid solvent left)
7. High-Energy, Ultra-Potent tinctures and extracts

High-Energy, Ultra-Potent

Certainly, the quality of the herbs used in a tincture (a highly concentrated liquid herbal formulation) is fundamental to its effectiveness, but it is by no means the only factor. How a tincture is made is of equal importance.

It has been known for centuries that if you time the "brewing" of a tincture to the phases of the moon, the resulting tincture is stronger. Specifically, if you start your tincture on the new moon and squeeze it on the full moon, it will be 10–15% stronger than an untimed tincture. This certainly sounds magical and mystical, particularly because no one has ever known why it works.

Nevertheless it has been demonstrated over and over again that those tinctures made in accordance with the phases of the moon are demonstrably stronger.

Incidentally, no commercial manufacturer "brews to the moon" because it takes too long (30 days). Instead, virtually all commercial manufacturers use a 3 or 4-day brewing process.

But recently, a remarkable discovery was made. While brainstorming one day

---

[1]The standardized commercial versions found in most stores, including health food stores.

with Ron Manwarren, the President of Royal Botanicals, I hit upon the actual principle behind "moon phase brewing." But even more importantly, I came up with an idea for how we could duplicate the "moon" effect when brewing tinctures—independent of the moon, many times stronger than the moon itself, and in less time. Ron was then able to take these ideas, add in a few of his own, and develop a process that incorporates this "Barron Effect™" into the brewing process—at a strength dozens of times stronger than the moon itself. The net result is herbal tinctures that are 50–100% stronger than anything the world has ever seen before. And not only are they stronger in the sense that the process produces more extract from a given amount of herbs, the tincture is also stronger in the sense that more biological components are now being extracted (components that were previously left behind by other extraction methods).

This process is not only effective for tinctures, but also allows for concentrates of significantly increased potency and effectiveness.

More Art Than Science

There's another issue that we need to deal with when talking about herbal medicine—another way in which herbs differ from drugs. At its best (most powerful, most effective, most healing), herbal medicine makes use of herbal formulations as opposed to single herbs. As in:

- You're anxious, take Kava
- You have a cold, take Echinacea

That's right out of traditional medicine. That's turning herbs into drugs. It's the least effective way to use herbs.

Herbal formulas, on the other hand, not only address particular symptoms, they also support the body as a whole. In addition, they make use of the synergistic effect inherent in many herbs. For example, many of the more powerful herbal formulations incorporate:

- Cayenne, not just because of its remarkable healing properties, but because cayenne is a potentiator for many other herbs, helping to energize them, to stimulate them, to "drive" them into the body.
- Lobelia, on the other hand, is a potentiator for "nerve-rebuilding" herbs, both stimulating ones such as Ginkgo and soothing ones such as St. John's Wort.

But only your more experienced herbalists are aware of these synergies and will know the proper proportions to use. Putting together effective herbal formulas is much more akin to art than science. To use the analogy of wine making again, the great herbalist is like the wine master. In the same way a wine expert can tell you the entire history and quality of wine with a single taste, a good herbalist can identify hundreds of herbs, and determine their quality, with a single taste. And just as no scientific equipment has ever come close to matching the taste buds of a wine expert, likewise no testing equipment comes close to matching the taste and sensitivity of the great herbalists.[1]

The bottom line is that Johnny-Come-Latelies to the herbal game are not going to have anything close to this level of expertise. They are merely throwing things together and using marketing muscle to convince you to buy their products. Does that mean that their products are useless? Not at all. But we're talking about the difference between Little League and Major League Baseball here. The great herbalists don't just cure colds; they cure cancer!

Is It That Important?

As we said at the beginning of this chapter, herbs are now coming into their own. The American public and even the American Medical Association are acknowledging that herbs can be beneficial. However, part of the paradigm that is being established is that "Yes, herbs can be helpful if you have a cold or a headache or want a little more mental clarity; but if you're really sick, you need real drugs." Bullpucky!!

You've been sold a bill of goods. Drug companies are spending millions and millions of dollars developing chemical knock-offs of herb-based phytochemicals. Tests consistently prove that the knock-offs are less effective, have serious side effects, and cost many many times more than the herb itself. Nevertheless, doctors prescribe the knock-off; people pay the inflated prices because their doctors prescribe it, and everybody suffers the consequences.

For example, when it comes to something serious like jacking up your immune system to fight cancer or repair damage to the pancreas or to help reverse diabetes—to put it simply—don't you want the natural formulation that's at 80–90% potency rather than the chemical knock-off that's at a "guaranteed" 25% potency and carries a whole series of side effects? In these situations, co-option can mean death.

General Recommendations

- Look for herbal formulations made from organic or wildcrafted herbs.
- Look for formulations designed by real herbalists.
- Look for herbal tinctures processed using the "Barron Effect".
- Look for (and expect) dramatic results.

---

[1]Standardization is a pale imitation of what a great herbalist can tell about herbal quality with a single taste.

CHAPTER 9

FREE RADICALS AND ANTIOXIDANTS

WHAT EXACTLY IS A FREE RADICAL?

A free radical is a cellular killer that wreaks havoc by damaging DNA, altering biochemical compounds, corroding cell membranes, and destroying cells outright. In this sense, a free radical can be thought of as an invader attacking the cells of your body. More technically, a free radical is a molecule that has lost one of its electrons and become highly unbalanced. It seeks to restore its balance by stealing a vital electron from another molecule.

Scientists now know that free radicals play a major role in the aging process as well as the onset of cancer, heart disease, stroke, arthritis, and possibly allergies and a host of other ailments. The link between free radicals and the "aging diseases" is the most important discovery since doctors learned that some illnesses are caused by germs.

In a very real sense, the free radical process in our bodies is much the same as the process that causes fuel to burn and oil to go rancid or an apple to turn brown if you slice it open and expose it to air. It is as though our bodies rust from the inside out—causing, among other things, dry, wrinkled skin. But wrinkles are the least of our problems. When the process gets really out of control, it can cause tumors, hardening of the arteries, and macular degeneration to name just a few.

The bottom line is that we can think of free radicals as ravenous molecular sharks—sharks so hungry that in little more than a millionth of a second, they can be making a frenzied attack on a healthy neighboring cellular molecule.

WHY ARE FREE RADICALS SO DEADLY?

A single free radical can destroy an enzyme, a protein molecule, a strand of DNA, or an entire cell. **Even worse, it can unleash, in a fraction of a second, a torrential chain reaction that produces a million or more additional killer free radicals.**

What Causes Free Radicals?

There are four primary sources of free radicals:

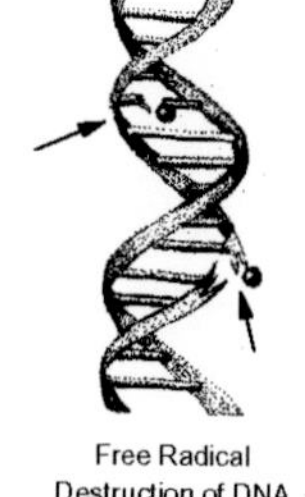
Free Radical Destruction of DNA

The Environment: Air pollution, cigarette smoke, smog, soot, automobile exhaust, toxic waste, pesticides, herbicides, ultraviolet light, background radiation, drugs, and even certain foods can all generate free radicals in the body.

Internal Production: Our bodies are constantly producing free radicals as a byproduct of normal metabolic functions.

Stress Factors: Aging, trauma, medications, disease, infection, and "stress" itself all accelerate the body's production of free radicals—oftentimes by a factor of eight times or more.

Chain Reactions: When a free radical steals an electron to balance itself out, it creates a new free radical in the molecule from which it stole the electron. In many cases the new free radical will seek to balance itself out by stealing an electron—and so on, and so on. And remember, even one free radical is capable of destroying an entire cell, or a strand of DNA.

Are All Free Radicals the Same?

There are many types of free radicals in the body. Four particularly nasty ones are:

1. **Superoxide radical:** This radical tries to steal its much-needed electron from the mitochondria of the cell. When mitochondria are destroyed, the cell loses its ability to convert food to energy. It dies.
2. **Hydroxyl radical:** This free radical attacks enzymes, proteins, and the unsaturated fats in cell membranes.
3. **Lipid peroxyl radical:** This radical unleashes a chain reaction of chemical events that can so totally compromise the cellular membrane that the cell bursts open, spews its contents, and dies.
4. **Singlet oxygen:** Not technically a free radical, this metabolite can nevertheless wreak havoc on the body.

Your body is constantly replacing and repairing free-radical damaged cells; but with the way we live and abuse ourselves, our bodies are bombarded with more free radicals than they can handle. By supplementing with antioxidants, we help our bodies keep up with the carnage. We can even get ahead of the game and reverse damage.

What Are Anitoxidants?

Antioxidants are compounds that render free radicals harmless and stop the chain-reaction formation of new free radicals.

Where Do They Come From?

There are three sources of antioxidants.

1. Several metabolic enzymes produced by the body are extremely effective antioxidant scavengers. Unfortunately, the body's ability to produce these enzymes fades dramatically in our late twenties.
2. Many foods and plants provide powerful antioxidants. Among these are Vitamins E and C, Beta Carotene, and the Proanthocyanidins (including Pycnogenol®).
3. Cutting edge research is continually uncovering new antioxidants.

What Are the Benefits of Antioxidants?

- Many scientists now believe that free radicals are the **major** villain in both aging and disease.
    - The amount of cells destroyed over the years by free radicals is enormous. Free radicals literally "eat away" the major organs of the body. Just one example: the size of a 25 year old's liver is often **twice** that of a person of 70.
- **The use of antioxidant supplements at a maintenance level may provide the ultimate defense against premature aging and a compromised immune system.**
- At therapeutic levels, antioxidants may actually play a significant role in **reversing many of the effects of aging and disease.**

General Recommendations

Over the years, I have formulated a number of antioxidant formulas for various companies. In fact, this is my specialty—the design of cutting edge nutritionals using standardized herbs and isolates. On the other hand, I have also become known as a strong advocate for the use of whole herbs and food complexes in all formulations. Why the apparent contradiction?

There is no question but that nature packages nutrients in food complexes, and that, in general, it is best to design supplements using only whole food complexes. Antioxidants, however, provide one of the few exceptions to that rule—as long as a few provisos are followed.

- The reason for the exception is that antioxidants are specialists, not generalists. No one antioxidant works on all free radicals and in every area of the body. For example, glutathione protects and repairs the liver, whereas Bilberry works to defend the eyes. The bottom line is that you need to combine a number of antioxidants in one supplement to offer an effective defense. (In fact, many antioxidants reinforce and/or recycle each other.) For maximum protection it is vital that you get an antioxidant complex that provides a full-spectrum defense. This is the only real defense against free radical devastation. For this reason, it is impossible to fit the variety you need (at adequate levels) into one supplement unless you use some standardized herbs and isolates.
- The trick is (1) to use only natural isolates—no synthetics, (2) to offer as complete a complex as you can even when using isolates, and (3) to make sure you **take advantage of the synergistic effect** that a number of the antioxidants share with each other.

The Ultimate Antioxidant

There is no such thing as an ultimate antioxidant, but look for a formula that pretty much matches the scope of the formula below and approximates the levels of each ingredient.

- **Beta carotene—5,620 IU**

  Carotenoids are phytonutrients that protect plants from damage caused by UV radiation and other environmental factors. In humans, they have been shown to inhibit the proliferation of various types of cancer cells such as those affecting the lungs, stomach, cervix, breast, bladder, and mouth. They also have been proven to protect against atherosclerosis, cataracts, macular degeneration, and other major degenerative disorders. The key carotenoids are beta carotene, alpha carotene, lycopene, and zeaxanthin.

  Probably the best known of the carotenoids, beta carotene, is converted by the body into vitamin A as needed to strengthen the immune system and promote healthy cell growth. In addition, beta carotene is a potent antioxidant, offering particular benefits to the immune system and the lungs. (Note: synthetic beta carotene is to be avoided at all costs and may not be required if provided in your daily multivitamin supplement.)

- **Alpha carotene—425 IU**

  Recent studies have shown that alpha carotene is one of the most powerful carotenoids and has a strong inhibitory effect on the proliferation of various types of cancer cells such as those affecting the lungs, stomach, cervix, breast, bladder, and mouth. It works by allowing normal cells to send growth-regulating signals to premalignant cells.

- **Lutein—8 mg**

  In addition to being a specific for the prevention of macular degeneration (lowering the risk by over 50%), lutein has also been shown to have strong anti-cancer properties. Its antioxidant effect is significantly enhanced by the presence of zeaxanthin and bilberry. When combined with vitamin C, these three antioxidants have been shown to significantly decrease the risk of cataracts.

- **Lycopene—6 mg**

  Derived primarily from tomatoes (cooked with olive oil, not raw), lycopene appears to be one of the best defenses against prostate cancer and bladder cancer. When used in conjunction with d-alpha-tocopherol vitamin E and green tea extract, studies indicate that it inhibits prostate cancer proliferation by some 90%.

- **Zeaxanthin—300 mcg**

  Lutein and zeaxanthin are both part of a group of carotenoids known as xanthophylls, which are extremely beneficial to the eyes and help significantly in the prevention of macular degeneration

- **Sodium Selenate—75 mcg**

  Selenium is synergistic with glutathione and catalase in helping to protect the integrity of cell membranes. It stops the growth of tumors, and it protects the liver.

  Specifically, low levels of selenium have been connected to death from heart disease, breast cancer, prostate cancer, colon cancer, and in fact, cancer of all kinds. Some studies have shown that selenium may be 50–100 times more powerful than any other anti-carcinogen known.

- **Sodium Citrate—300 mg**

  Revitalizes collagen and elastin fibers to rejuvenate the skin and the collagen-rich connective tissue of the arterial walls.

- **N-Acetyl-Cysteine (NAC)—225 mg**

  One of the keys to a healthy immune system is maintaining high levels of glutathione in the body. Unfortunately, supplementing with glutathione doesn't really help. Fortunately, there are alternatives. Supplementation with N-acetyl-cysteine (NAC) has been proven to substantially raise the body's glutathione levels. In addition, NAC supplementation is mandatory for all smokers and big-city dwellers as it protects against toxic aldehydes that enter the body through cigarette smoke and pollution.

- **L-Methionine—225 mg**

  An essential sulfur amino acid, methionine is a powerful antioxidant and liver detoxifier—where it assists in the normal detoxification processes. As an antioxidant, it provides powerful protection in the colon. And finally, methionine is involved in the synthesis of choline, adrenaline, lecithin, and B12, and it works as a powerful SAMe precursor.

- **Quercetin—180 mg**

  Quercetin is one of the class of antioxidants known as bioflavonoids. A prime role of quercetin is to protect the integrity of cell walls from free radical damage. In addition, quercetin prevents the release of histamines into the bloodstream, thereby helping to control food and pollen allergies.

- **Gingko biloba—180 mg (24/6%)**

  Known as the brain antioxidant, gingko has been shown to increase brain functionality, which makes it useful in helping to improve concentration and memory. This makes it a specific for Alzheimer's, where it has the added benefit of helping to significantly reduce depression.

  In addition, gingko oxygenates the blood, increases circulation, and strengthens blood vessels. And finally, its anti-inflammatory, lung-relaxant properties have proven useful in the treatment of asthma, where it eases coughing and reduces tissue inflammation.

- **Curcumin—120 mg**

  Curcumin is what gives turmeric its yellow color. Studies have shown that it can inhibit colon cancer cells by some 96% in a matter of hours. It also appears to have great potential in countering the effects of prostate cancer and breast cancer. In a sense, curcumin can be thought of as natural chemotherapy—with the ability to selectively kill cancer cells, while at the same time leaving normal cells alone. Note: Curcumin and green tea strongly reinforce each other.

- **Green tea extract—120 mg (83%)**

  Green tea antioxidants are of the same family as grape seed and pine bark extracts. They are polyphenols, chief of which are the flavonoids called proanthocyanidins. In green tea, the main proanthocyanidins are the catechins, and the most powerful of the catechins is Epigallocatechin Gallate (EGCG), found in the highest concentration in green tea.

Green tea works to prevent tumors from developing the blood vessels they need to survive. It has been shown to inhibit metastasis. And it is the first known natural telomerase inhibitor. That is to say, it eliminates the "immortality" of cancer cells which is their trademark and which makes them so deadly. Green tea is particularly effective in destroying the causes of leukemia, prostate cancer, and breast cancer.

And the benefits of green tea don't stop there. It has also been shown to be effective in regulating blood sugar, reducing triglycerides and in reversing the ravages of heart disease. (Incidentally, the Japanese, who drink large amounts of green tea, have some of the lowest rates of cardiovascular disease in the world.)

Green tea seems to be able to almost totally prevent cancer causing DNA damage in smokers—a possible explanation as to why the Japanese, who are among the world's heaviest smokers, have such a low incidence of lung cancer.

And finally, green tea has great benefits for the brain as well, serving as an effective MAO inhibitor, protecting against brain-cell death from glucose oxidase, overproduction of nitric oxide, and lowering the amount of free iron reaching the brain (a bad thing). The net result is that there are strong indications that green tea extract may play a major role in protecting against both Parkinson's and Alzheimer's disease.

Note: if you drink green tea, adding cream or milk to the tea seems to destroy all antioxidant benefits.

- **Bilberry—120 mg (25%)**

The anthocyanosides found in bilberry are known for their ability to help nourish and repair the tiny capillaries within the eye. In addition, the bilberry bioflavonoids are beneficial to the connective tissue that lines blood vessels and binds ligaments throughout the body.

- **Alpha lipoic acid—100 mg**

Sometimes called the "Mother" antioxidant, alpha lipoic acid (ALA) plays a major role in helping recycle vitamins E and C so that they can be used over and over again by your body. In its own right, ALA is one of the main boosters of glutathione levels in body cells, and is one of the key co-factors involved in generating energy in the cells mitochondria. And finally, ALA has also been shown to significantly rejuvenate the cognitive skills of people as they age.

- **SOD—75 mg**

Superoxide dismutase (SOD) works along with glutathione to neutralize reactive oxygen molecules in the body. SOD specifically targets the superoxide radical, which, as we discussed earlier, attacks cell mitochondria. When mitochondria are destroyed, the cell loses its ability to convert food to energy. It dies. SOD also works in the cytoplasm of the cell to prevent the hydroxyl radical from attacking enzymes, proteins, and the unsaturated fats in cell membranes.

- **Tocotrienols—75 mg**

  Derived from rice bran or palm oil, tocotrienols are a unique vitamin E fraction that is 40 times more powerful than standard vitamin E. Tocotrienols are rich in the gamma tocopherol fraction of vitamin E that strongly inhibits both the estrogen-responsive and the non-estrogen responsive breast cancer cells.

- **Grape skin extract—60 mg**

  For several years, grape seed extract was all the rage. As it turns out, grape **skin** extract, also called Resveratrol, is equally powerful. In controlled studies, Resveratrol has been shown to reduce skin cancer tumors by up to 98%, to stop production of leukemia cells. In addition, it works as a Cox inhibitor, thus halting the spread of cancer throughout the body.

- **Grape seed extract—60 mg (84-93%)**

  Similar to green tea, the active ingredients in grape seed extract are the proanthocyanidins (but in a different combination and ratio). The importance of the proanthocyanidins in grape seed extract is that they are water soluble and highly bio-available. Above all else, grape seed extract is known as a defender of the circulatory system. It improves peripheral circulation, revives declining capillary activity by up to 140%, and increases vascular response by some 82%. It repairs varicose veins and aids in the prevention of bruising.

  In addition, grape seed extract is synergistic with vitamin C, vastly increasing vitamin C activity and strengthening collagen activity—including in the connective tissue of the arterial wall and the skin.

- **Chaparral extract—375 mcg**

  The active antioxidant in Chaparral, a lignan called Nordihydroguaiaretic Acid (NDGA), has been shown to specifically target virtually all forms of herpes virus—and has been shown to be up to 97.5% effective. It also is an effective counter to radiation induced free radical damage. And there are strong indications it is an effective aid in the prevention of Alzheimer's and rheumatoid arthritis.

- **Catalase—300 mcg**

  Glutathione perioxidase, superoxide dismutase, and catalase are the primary three enzymes produced in the body as an antioxidant defense. Catalase is a specific for protection against tumors.

OTHER ANTIOXIDANTS

There are other antioxidants that are well worth taking, but because of the quantity needed to be effective, make no sense to include as part of an overall formula. These include:

- **Red Raspberry Ellagitannins**

  Scientific studies have proven that supplementation with 40 mg per day of red raspberry ellagitannins prevents the development of cancer cells. At low concentrations, it slows the growth of cancer cells; at higher concentrations, it tells cancer cells to kill themselves.

- **L-Carnosine**

  L-carnosine is a naturally occurring combination of two amino acids, alanine and histadine that can actually **reverse** the signs of aging. It works as an antioxidant to protect cellular protein from attack by carbonyl groups and prevents the oxidation of sugars in the body. Supplementation with carnosine represents one of the most powerful things you can do to hold back the ravages of old age.

- **Vitamin E**

  In addition to protecting the cardiovascular system, vitamin E is particularly effective in reducing the incidence and mortality of prostate cancer. 400 IU a day of all-natural unesterified mixed tocopherols and tocotrienols, containing no vegetable oil that can go rancid, is recommended.

- **Vitamin C**

  The antioxidant benefits of vitamin C are invaluable. The trick is that almost all of the vitamin C sold today is virtually unusable by the body. You need 500–1,000 mg of vitamin C a day—but it must be in a "living-food matrix," that is bound to food so your body can use it.

- **Methylation**

  Although technically not a free radical problem, the results of methylation (the exchange of methyl groups in the body) has similar effects. As we age, our body's ability to provide methyl donor groups declines. The bottom line is that everyone should be on a supplement to prevent homocysteine damage to the cardiovascular system, cancer, DNA damage, and deterioration of the brain. S-adenosylmethionine, also known as SAMe is a popular alternative. But a less expensive choice is to purchase at any discount health store a formula that contains 500 mg of trimethylglycine, 50 mg of B-6, 800 mcg of folic acid, 500 mcg of B-12 (best in the form of methylcobalamine, if you can find it).

Foods

Certain foods are high in antioxidants and should be a regular part of the diet. In fact, the US Department of Agriculture recently rated a large number of foods according to their Oxygen Radical Absorbence Capacity. The higher the number, the more powerful the antioxidant value. All ratings were based on 3½ ounce of the tested food. As a reference, carrots (high in the carotenoids) had a 207 rating.

- **Broccoli florets, Brussels sprouts, Raw spinach, and Kale**

  Broccoli carries a rating of 890, brussels sprouts 980, spinach 1,260, and kale 1,770. Be aware that these foods contain other phytonutrients that go well beyond their antioxidant value.

- **Strawberries, Blueberries, and Raisins**

  Strawberries at 1,540, blueberries at 2,400, and raisins at 2,830, all rate high.

- **Prunes**

  Whoa! The lowly prune is top rated at 5,770. Eat prunes daily!

- **Soy Products**

  Although not antioxidants, genistein and the other isoflavones in soy nevertheless reduce the risk of many kinds of cancer, stimulate bone formation, protect the kidneys, and inhibit deterioration of the cardiovascular system. Regular consumption of soy products makes sense for most people—but not for children, and particularly not for infants, because of the high level of phytoestrogens in soy.

Chapter 10

Balancing Hormone Levels in the Body

In a perfect world, there would be no need to address this aspect of health at all, but the world we live in is far from perfect. Again, diet, stress, and environmental factors are constantly working to throw our bodies out of balance. Specifically, we need to address the following problem areas.

- Due to exposure to chemical estrogens omnipresent in our food, water, and air, the vast majority of men and women already suffer the effects of estrogen dominance by the time they are in their early 30s.
- Again due to diet and lifestyle, most men and women find that their testosterone has become "unavailable" by the time they are in their early 30s. For men, that problem is compounded by the fact that what testosterone they do have is being converted into dihydrotestosterone, which leads to prostate enlargement and cancer.

For years, I have been leery of recommending the use of formulas that modify the body's hormonal balance, and certainly the misuse of hormone altering formulas by athletes and medical doctors in the last decade has not helped change that point of view.

Nevertheless, once you throw out all of the preconceptions and look at the issue objectively (and look at the real results—short and long term), the case for **selectively** altering your hormonal balance becomes compelling—with a few caveats:

- Only selected hormones should be "adjusted" without a doctor's guidance.
- Use only natural hormones (or hormones that are chemically **identical** to the natural hormone).
  - Note: Hormones are produced from many different sources. Some are derived from animals; some from plants; some are created in laboratories; and some are created through changing the DNA of bacteria or single-celled plants so that they produce the desired hormone. As it turns out, for hormones, the source is not the real question. The real question is: Is the hormone a perfect match for the hormone in our bodies? As we will soon see for estrogen and progesterone, things are not always what they seem.

- Use only therapeutic or homeopathic doses. Never, ever use pharmacological doses[1] without a doctor's guidance.

Estrogen and Progesterone

Vital Information for Women (And Men)

Every woman between the ages of 13 and 117 needs to seriously consider supplementation with a natural progesterone creme.

Why? Because virtually every woman who lives in an industrialized country (the United States, in particular) is at high risk of estrogen dominance because of exposure to xenoestrogens. Xenoestrogens, which are mostly petroleum-based synthetic estrogens, are now present in massive amounts in our food chain, water supply, and environment.

At one time, our diets afforded some protection. Fruits and grains and vegetables (in their natural state) provide low-action phytoestrogens for the body. These low-action estrogens fill the body's estrogen receptor sites—making them unavailable for use by the more potent estrogens—both natural and synthetic. Unfortunately, today's diets are dominated by processed foods, which are stripped of these beneficial phytoestrogens. The net result is that virtually all of the body's receptor sites are ready and waiting for the far more intense estrogens.

Some high-potency estrogens (such as estrone and estradiol) are produced by the body itself. But far and away, the greatest problem comes from the powerful and destructive petrochemical-based xenoestrogens. Not only are these xenoestrogens omnipresent, they are considerably more potent than estrogen made by the ovaries—**some even potent in amounts as small as a billionth of a gram.**

Before we proceed, it is important to understand what role estrogen plays in the body. In addition to promoting the growth of female characteristics at puberty, the estrogen hormones also promote cell growth. It is the estrogens, for example, that stimulate the buildup of tissue and blood in the uterus at the start of the menstrual cycle. The problem comes when high levels of estrogen (natural and synthetic) are unopposed by sufficient amounts of natural progesterone, which leads to continuous, unrestrained cell stimulation. Problems that can occur include:

- Excess estrogen is the only known cause of endometrial cancer.
- Increased risk of breast cancer.
- Loss of bone mass.

---

[1]Therapeutic doses mimic the amount of hormone your body normally produces. Pharmacological (or medicinal doses) are substantially higher than therapeutic doses—and are often accompanied by significant side effects.

- Increased risk of autoimmune disorders such as lupus.
- Fibrocystic breasts.
- Fibroid tumors.
- Depression and irritability.
- PMS symptoms such as cramping and bloating—in addition to depression and irritability.
- Menopausal symptoms such as hot flashes and night sweats—again, in addition to depression and irritability.
- Decreased sex drive.
- Increased body hair and thinning of scalp hair.
- Migraine headaches.
- Impaired thyroid function, including Grave's disease.
- Increased body fat.
- Increased blood clotting.
- Impaired blood sugar control.
- The astounding acceleration of puberty in young girls from an average age of 14 to 15, to now as young as 9 or 10. (This represents a speed up of as much as ⅓ sooner in their lives and has frightening implications for long-term health.)
- And, finally, xenoestrogens have been strongly implicated in declining male sperm production and the increase in the rates of testicular cancer and prostate cancer.

What's the Answer?

Once we understand the problem, it is easy to see that for the vast majority of women, hormone replacement therapy with conjugated estrogens such as Premarin® is not the answer. It very well may be a major contributor to the problem.

Most people are not aware that Premarin® is actually derived from horse urine. Hence the name: **Pre**gnant **mar**e ur**in**e. This is not a problem in itself, but it does **lead** to three significant problems.

1. First, and **most important:** there is no estriol in Premarin®, only estrone and estradiol. Why is this so significant? Because research has shown that the average ratio of serum estrogen in the female body is 90% estriol, 7%

estradiol, and 3% estrone. This takes on particular importance when one notes that both estrone and estradiol are pro-carcinogenic, whereas estriol is anti-carcinogenic. So why in the world would you want to use an estrogen supplement that has only the pro-carcinogenic estrogens, and not one single drop of the anti-carcinogenic estrogen that normally represents 90% of the body's total? The bottom line is that in those cases where estrogen supplementation is warranted, demand either "true triple estrogen" from your doctor and insist that it be in a ratio similar to the 90-7-3 shown above or use pure estriol.

2. Second, there are over a **dozen** different estrogens in Premarin®. As you may remember from our earlier discussion of estrogen, there are only three estrogens in the human body: estrone, estradiol, and estriol. Only two of those are present in Premarin®: estrone and estradiol. That means that there are a whole bunch of estrogens in Premarin® that have nothing to do with the human body. They are specifically designed for horses. (Keep in mind that the Latin word for horse is *equs* from which comes equestrian.) Some of these include equilin, 17 alpha-dihydroequilin, and equilenin. Another way of looking at it is that those "extra" estrogens are specifically designed to make you gallop and whinny.

3. Third, the process of producing Premarin® is inherently cruel. The mares are kept in tiny pens to eliminate movement. They are kept constantly pregnant. And they are kept constantly catheterized. The process is so stressful that the average life expectancy of these animals is less than half that of a normal horse. And of course the foals are not needed, so they are destroyed.

You really have to wonder why more doctors don't ask, "If estrogen dominance got you there in the first place, then why in the world would you want to be adding a powerful estrogen complex made from horse urine to your body?" Of course you wouldn't. And yet, conjugated estrogen is the most frequently prescribed drug in America. Consider the following scenario—one that millions of women have already lived through.

> One day you notice minor symptoms such as a sudden gain in weight or a disruption in sleep patterns or a decreased sex drive. You go for a check-up and receive a prescription for estrogen. As instructed, you take your daily dose of horse urine, but the symptoms get steadily worse. You're told to increase your dosage. Which you do. But the symptoms continue to get worse, and over time become alarming, since they now include problems such as irregular cycles, heavy clotting, or excessive bleeding. An examination of your uterus reveals significant abnormality. You are told your uterus is precancerous. Your hysterectomy is scheduled; your uterus is removed.

This is absolutely and totally unacceptable. Every woman should be furious!

The only **natural** balancer to excessive estrogen in the body is **natural** progesterone—not more estrogen. This has been clearly detailed in books such as *What Your Doctor May Not Tell You About Menopause,* by Dr. John R. Lee. Natural progesterone is the only known substance that mitigates virtually all of the problems associated with estrogen dominance, and with virtually no side effects of its own.

But what about the synthetic "progesterones" (such as Provera) that your doctor recommends? Progesterone is a natural substance, and as such cannot be patented. The pharmaceutical companies, therefore, have to modify it slightly. They literally create a new molecule, called medroxyprogesterone—that does not exist in nature—in order to take out a patent. This "slightly" modified artificial progesterone is what most doctors prescribe. What effect does slight modification have?

Consider the fact that the testosterone molecule and the estrone molecule are virtually identical—except for the fact that the positions of the oxygen atom and the OH atoms change places. This slight "modification," however, happens to be enough so that one hormone makes men...and the other women.

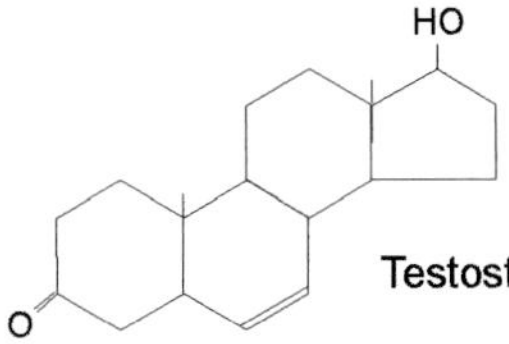

HO
O
Testosterone

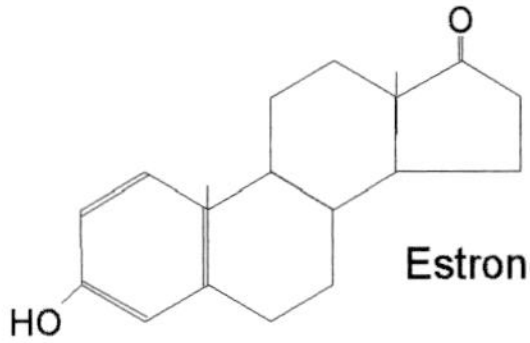

O
HO
Estrone

Even closer is the similarity between DHEA and estrone. The molecules are actually identical except for the location of some of the double bonds between carbon atoms. You cannot get closer. And yet the function of DHEA and estrone could not be more different.

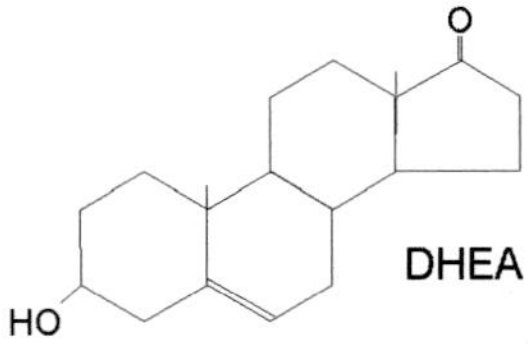

O
HO
DHEA

And now look at the difference between natural progesterone and Provera.

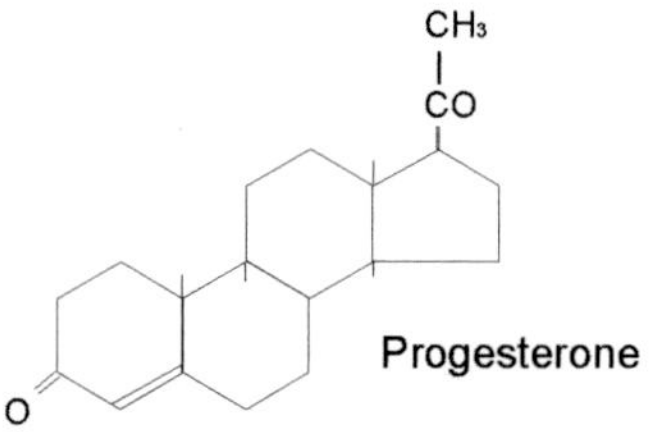

CH_3
CO
O
Progesterone

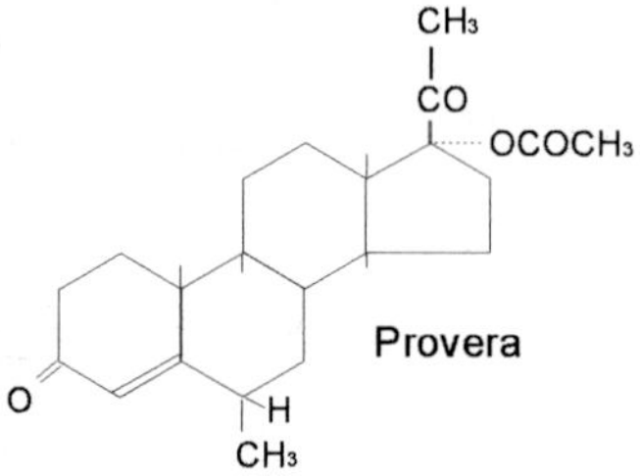

CH_3
CO
$OCOCH_3$
O
H
CH_3
Provera

The bottom line is that Provera is not natural. It's a synthetic form of progesterone that carries a whole range of serious side effects. A small sampling of these side effects, as listed in the *Physician's Desk Reference,* includes:

- Depression
- Birth defects
- Increased body hair
- Acne
- Risk of embolism
- Decreased glucose tolerance
- Allergic reactions

Now, in exchange for these significant side effects, Provera does offer some protection against endometrial cancer and **a very modest increase** in bone formation.

Natural Progesterone

On the other hand, supplementation with natural progesterone has **no** known side effects. It is best utilized by the body when administered transdermally with a skin cream that contains approximately 500 milligrams per ounce of natural progesterone and offers the following potential health benefits.

- According to Dr. John R. Lee, the author of *What Your Doctor May Not Tell You About Menopause,* natural progesterone may significantly improve bone formation—by as much as 15%–35%. (Understand, this is unique to natural progesterone. Estrogen supplementation does not increase bone formation; it merely slows the rate of loss for a 5-year period around the time of menopause. And manmade progestin only mildly increases bone formation. **If you are worried about osteoporosis, there is only one substance known that significantly improves bone formation—and that's natural progesterone.)**

- Increased progesterone levels in the body may help to protect against endometrial cancer.
- They may also help protect against breast cancer.
- In addition, supplementation with natural progesterone can help relieve symptoms of PMS.
- Relieve symptoms of menopause.
- Normalize libido.
- Improve the body-fat profile.
- Improve sleep patterns.
- And help relieve migraine headaches.

The bottom line is that every woman living in the industrialized world should seriously consider supplementation with natural progesterone.

If you decide to begin a regimen of natural progesterone supplementation, look for a premium quality balancing cream that contains a minimum of 500 milligrams per ounce (the amount recommended by Dr. Lee) of 100% pure, USP grade progesterone, naturally derived from soybeans. Look for a natural vegetarian formula that uses no artificial or synthetically derived fragrances, parabens or preservatives. Look for a formula that uses all natural oils and an enhanced liposome delivery system to help move the progesterone through the skin. And finally, look for a formula that uses only full-profile **organic** wild yam.

Whether you're still going through your menstrual cycles (or whether you're pre-menopausal, menopausal, or post-menopausal), you need to seriously consider supplementation. The benefits are extraordinary; the risks virtually nonexistent. And the risks of not supplementing potentially include an increased risk of breast cancer, endometrial cancer, and osteoporosis—to reiterate just a few.

And as for Men

As we've already mentioned in the preceding paragraphs, men too are exposed to the effects of xenoestrogens. In addition, as their testosterone levels drop with age (see next section), there is, in many cases, a concomitant rise in estradiol levels—the major reason that many older men develop breasts.

Just as with women, estradiol stimulates cell growth[1] in men too and is potentially cancerous. **This is one of the main factors involved in the dramatically increased incidence of prostrate cancer.** In other words, any man over 30 years old would be well advised to supplement with a natural progesterone cream.

---

[1]Estradiol stimulates the BCL2 gene, which is the gene responsible for stopping cell death. What at first glance sounds like a positive, is, upon closer inspection, not. When cell death in prostate tissue, for example, is blocked, cell growth continues unabated, becoming a major contributing factor in the enlargement of the prostate and the development of prostate cancer.

Testosterone

A growing body of evidence suggests that testosterone levels drop as much as 40% in men between their early 40s and early 70s. And for 10 to 15 percent of all men, those levels will dip below normal even as early as their 30s if there is stress, depression, personal life changes or medications. This in turn causes a decrease, not only in sexual desire and performance, but in the competitive drive to succeed and accomplish in life. In women, excessive estrogen in the body causes a reduction in testosterone levels, which leads to a similar decline in sexual desire and performance and a similar reduction in "life drive."

Wild Oats and Nettles

As we've just discussed, available testosterone levels tend to diminish with age. Adequate testosterone levels are essential in sexual functioning and "life drive" for both sexes. Women, for example, with high testosterone levels have more sex, increased libido, more orgasms, and tighter bonds with their mates.

Interestingly enough, in a 1986 clinical study, it was documented that it's not actual testosterone production that decreases as people age. What happens is that it's the amount of **free circulating** testosterone that decreases—as more and more of it gets bound to albumin and becomes unavailable for the body's use. These changes appear to begin by middle age and happen through a natural chemical process called "sex-hormone-binding-globulin" or "SHBG".

The problem is that bound testosterone is not nearly as effective as free testosterone in stimulating the sex and "life drive" centers in the brain. **Avena sativa (green oats) and urtica dioica (nettles) easily travel throughout the body and free up testosterone—thus increasing desire.** In studies, these two herbs

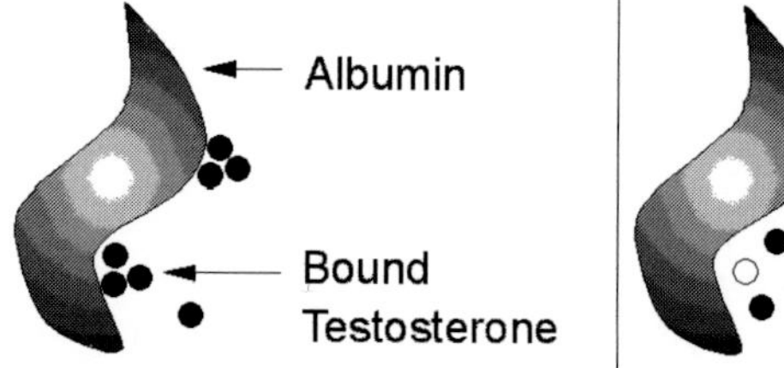

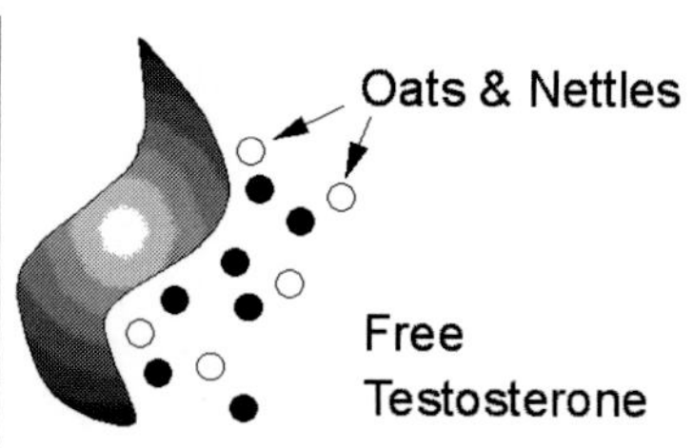

increased free testosterone levels an astounding 105% on average!

Green oats and nettles work naturally with the body to enhance sexual desire, sensation, and performance in both men and women. The effect on human sexual appetite is powerful. Both men and women can feel a boost in sexual desire—sometimes after only a few hours. Both men and women experience an increase in frequency of orgasms while taking wild oats and nettles, while many women experience a dramatic 68% increase in multiple orgasms. Men also reported multiple orgasms while taking the wild oats and nettles combination.

Green oats and wild nettles also work naturally to enhance the "life drive," that competitive drive in both men and women to succeed and accomplish in life.

Human Growth Hormone

Why HGH?

The rejuvenating powers of Growth Hormone are no secret to the wealthy. Unfortunately, for the last 30 years, GH has been available only from doctors, required two injections a day, and cost approximately a thousand dollars a month. Recently, however, several alternatives for the rest of us have become available. And while I could never recommend the injections (for a variety of reasons), I can endorse the alternatives.

Many claims are made for the effects of Growth Hormone—some bordering on claims of "almost" immortality and "almost" eternal youth. Would that it were so! Although the effects are more subtle, for most people, than pronounced, they are nevertheless wide ranging, and include things such as:

- 14.4% loss of fat on average after 6 months without dieting
- Elimination of cellulite
- Higher energy levels
- Enhanced sexual performance
- Superior immune function
- Greater cardiac output
- Hair regrowth
- Regrowth of heart, liver, spleen, kidneys,and other organs that shrink with age
- Improved cholesterol profile, with higher HDL, and lower LDL
- Lowered blood pressure
- Increased exercise performance
- Better kidney function
- Stronger bones
- Faster wound healing
- Younger, tighter, thicker skin

Which HGH?

First of all, you can no longer actually buy true Human Growth Hormone. Technically, only actual growth hormone taken from human beings can be called Human Growth Hormone. And in fact, 30 years ago, that was the sole source of Growth Hormone—human cadavers, that is. But that was abandoned when it turned out that growth hormone taken from people had a major downside (in addition to cost)—and that was that it occasionally caused the human equivalent of mad cow disease. Not good, as they say.

Fortunately, at around the same time it was determined that true Human Growth Hormone was not an acceptable alternative, recombinant DNA technology came into its own. The bottom line is that scientists learned how to alter the DNA of a single-cell yeast plant so that it would produce large amounts of Growth Hormone (molecularly, absolutely identical to real Human Growth Hormone) safely and inexpensively. Because this growth hormone is identical to HGH, people often use the terms Growth Hormone and Human Growth Hormone interchangeably. Technically, however, it should be referred to as a plant-based Growth Hormone and not Human Growth Hormone. Many companies deliberately try and cross this line.

Anyway, given that there now existed a good, inexpensive source of Growth Hormone, another problem remained. It turns out that the Growth Hormone molecule is so large (containing 191 amino acids) that it could not be absorbed orally. That meant it could only be administered by injection. This, of course, required a doctor and was very expensive—costing between $1,000 and $1,800 a month.[1]

The only alternatives to this for years have been the amino acid–based precursor formulas (also called secretagogues). Although not as powerful as HGH injections, these formulas can be quite effective (provided your pituitary is still functioning well) and carry none of the downside of the injections.

Within the last two years, two alternatives have appeared on the market that actually use real Growth Hormone (the plant-based variety). One is homeopathic GH. This makes use of real GH, diluted down to homeopathic levels. The jury is still out on homeopathic HGH, but the early indications are that it works at least as well as the secretagogues.

And recently, a new form of GH that can be absorbed orally has been introduced. This again works as well as a secretogogue for most people. Its advantage is that this version will work for those few whose pituitaries are dead and no longer capable of producing HGH, whereas a secreatogogue will not. Its downside is cost, as it is the most expensive of the alternatives (but still far less costly than the injections).

Let me digress for a moment and explain exactly how GH works. First of all, as we detailed in our discussion of progesterone, it is important to understand that hormones are the body's chemical messenger system. They tell the body what to do and when. Adrenaline, for example, is produced in the adrenal glands, but serves to tell the heart to speed up and the blood vessels to narrow in times of stress. HGH, on the other hand is produced in the pituitary gland. It is released in a series of 9-24 microscopic "pulses" throughout the day (mostly in the evening), and it signals a number of body functions relative to aging

---

[1]Because of the cost involved, growth hormone injections became known as the secret youth formula of movie stars and the very rich.

and the production of other hormones such as DHEA and Melatonin and various parts of the endocrine system, including the hypothalamus (considered to be the master gland). Interestingly enough, the release of GH at "pulse" levels stimulates the pituitary to produce even more GH. However, it's most important function is telling the liver to produce Insulin-like Growth Factor (IGF-1). That's the main key to anti-aging. Specifically, the benefits of HGH can be measured in terms of how much it increases the body's production of IGF-1.[1] Any number above 20% starts to be significant in terms of effectiveness for anti-aging.

Most of the formulas on the market will increase IGF-1 levels by a minimum of 20%—some even approaching 100%.[2] Keep in mind, however, that one 30-minute aerobic session can easily increase IGF-1 levels by a good 100%, and a solid session of weight training can increase levels by an incredible 400–800%.

DHEA

In animal studies, DHEA supplementation bordered on the miraculous. It seemed to:

- Extend life by 50%
- Protect against heart disease, cancer, autoimmune diseases, obesity, and diabetes
- Boost the immune system
- Reverse the effects of stress

The reality turned out to be somewhat less.

I am not a big fan of DHEA supplementation (at least without a blood

---

[1] There is some concern that HGH (because it increases IGF-1 levels in the body) may increase the risk of prostate cancer. This is based on three observations: a couple of in vitro studies that showed IGF-1 may stimulate tumor cell growth, a study out of the Harvard School of Public Health that equated high levels of IGF-1 with increased risk of prostate cancer, and the fact that "giants" (who are, in fact, giants because of abnormally high HGH levels) have a higher risk of cancer. A simple reality check, however, calls these observations into question. First, the reality is that both HGH and IGF-1 levels decline as we age. The incidence of prostate cancer, on the other hand, increases as these levels decline—the exact opposite of the expressed concern. In addition, in numerous studies with thousands and thousands of patients receiving large amounts of HGH supplementation through injection over many years, there was no observed increase in prostate cancer. In fact, based on real-life observation, there is evidence to the contrary, that HGH supplementation may actually reduce the risk of prostate cancer.

[2] Injections, which work directly on the liver (almost like a massive "pulse," can increase IGF-1 production by 20-40%. (A downside to injections, in addition to cost, is that they can give too much GH to the body, shock the body, and can stop the pituitary from producing its own GH. This may explain why injectable GH produces more immediate results, yet ultimately results in a plateau.)

workup) for several reasons. First of all, the oral DHEA commonly used[1] is composed of particles that are too big to be directly used by the body; therefore, it has to be sent to the liver to be broken down. Unfortunately, since the liver is unaccustomed to receiving DHEA in this form, it ends up converting most of it into androgens (sex hormones). It is these androgens that can cause the growth of facial hair in women and may contribute to prostate disorders in men.[2] The second problem with standard oral DHEA supplementation is that there is strong evidence it reduces the body's own production of DHEA. And finally, DHEA supplementation (usually in doses greater than 10 mg a day) is often accompanied by side effects that include:

- Acne and excessive oiliness
- Growth of face and body hair in women
- Irritability or mood changes
- Overstimulation and insomnia

7-Keto

As we mentioned earlier, the oral DHEA commonly available is composed of particles that are too big to be directly used; therefore, it is sent to the liver, which ends up converting most of it into androgens. What's left is converted into 7-Keto DHEA, the useful portion. Well, now a new form of DHEA is available, 7-Keto DHEA. It seems that 7-Keto may provide most of the benefits of regular DHEA, but since it can't be converted to active androgens (e.g., testosterone and estrogen), it should prove to be much safer and have minimal side effects.The only downside is that 7-Keto is brand new and there have been no substantial clinicals to support it. All in all though, if you're looking to supplement with DHEA, 7-Keto probably makes the most sense. Note: Many people use supplements containing Mexican Wild Yam (Discorea villosa) as a DHEA supplement. The theory is that Wild Yam contains diosgenin, a DHEA precursor, that your body uses to produce its own DHEA. Unfortunately, there

---

[1] The DHEA commonly available as a supplement is not the same as that used in studies.

[2] There has been a lot of debate as to whether DHEA contributes to prostate problems or not. I think that, as with HGH, once you step back, you see that most of the debate makes no sense. The argument is that since DHEA can be converted into testosterone and dihydrotestosterone, hormones that are believed to stimulate prostate tissue, it has also been proposed that DHEA is counterproductive in those who have prostate gland enlargement or prostate tumors. But actual experience does not support that conclusion. The only case I have heard of that showed a definite link was one in which the patient was receiving doses of DHEA that reached 700 mg a day. That's many many times the 2-50 mg a day dose that makes any sense. There is evidence that at low dosage levels DHEA works to block androgen receptor sites in the body—making them unavailable to the more potent androgens—thus serving to protect your prostate.

is no evidence that, in fact, your body converts any Wild Yam into DHEA. All benefits related to Wild Yam appear to be from its phytoestrogen effect.

PREGNENOLONE

Pregnenolone is the ultimate hormone precursor. Virtually every hormone in the body can be produced by your body, as required, from pregnenolone. Again, as with all of the other hormones that we've talked about in this chapter, pregnenolone levels decline precipitously as you get older.

The prime benefit of pregnenolone is that it helps balance out your other hormone levels as required. In addition, though, it does provide specific benefits, such as:

- Extremely powerful memory enhancement and improved cognitive performance
- Supports the adrenals
- A strong antifatigue agent
- Of significant benefit in rheumatologic and connective tissue disorders such as rheumatism, osteoarthritis, scleroderma, psoriasis, lupus, and spondylitis
- Repair of the myelin sheath structure
- Improved immunity
- Reduced PMS and menopausal symptoms
- And it just makes you "feel" really good

Use of pregnenolone has shown no serious side effects even at very high doses of up to 700 mg. However, at the high dosage level, there has been some occurance of minor side effects, including overstimulation and insomnia, irritability, anger or anxiety, acne, and headaches.

MELATONIN

Melatonin is a natural hormone made in the pineal gland, a pea-sized gland located in the brain. Since its first discovery in 1958, melatonin has been studied extensively and has been shown to be widely beneficial to the body. As with all of the other hormones we're discussing, melatonin levels decline significantly as we age. An interesting note on melatonin. The trigger for production of melatonin is darkness—total darkness.[1] Any light in the room will inhibit production of your body's melatonin. Today, however, living in a world with night-lights in the bedroom, or streetlights sneaking through the window, we actually have an epidemic of people with insufficient melatonin production, even at a very young age. Now here's the really interesting part. The problem doesn't just come from light falling on our eyes while we sleep, but from light falling on any part of the body. Even if you wear an eye-mask, so that you are in total darkness, if light is falling on your arms or chest or feet, that's enough to stop melatonin production.

The benefits of supplementation include:

- Better Sleep
  - Lowered levels of nighttime melatonin reduce the quality of sleep resulting in the need for more sleep. If your pineal gland does not produce adequate melatonin early enough in the evening, both the quality and quantity of your sleep may suffer. Lack of melatonin may make it difficult for you to fall asleep, or may cause you to wake up too soon. Too much melatonin and you will feel yourself feeling exhausted, or "drugged" throughout the day. If secretion does not continue, you may wake up too soon. By taking melatonin instead of other so-called sleeping aids, rapid eye movement sleep (REM=dreaming) is not suppressed nor does it induce "hangover" effects when used as directed.
- Enhanced Immune Function
  - Many people report that supplementation with melatonin has significantly reduced their incidence of colds and infections. The exact way in which melatonin affects the immune system is not known. However, since much of the activity of the immune system takes place at night, some researchers have proposed that melatonin interacts with the immune system during sleep, helping to buffer the adverse effects of stress on the immune system.[2]
- Powerful Antioxidant Capabilities
  - Melatonin is one of the most powerful antioxidants produced in the body. In addition, since it is both water and fat soluble, melatonin can reach almost every single cell in the body. On the down side, however, since it cannot store in the body, it must be replenished daily. This would normally not be a problem, except for the fact, as we've already mentioned, that

---

[1]Without artificial light we would normally be in total darkness from 8–12 hours a night, producing melatonin during all of those hours. Living in a city or suburban area may cut the hours of total darkness to 0–6, depending on how light tight the bedroom is.

[2]It has been proposed by some that the increased incidence of cancer we are seeing is partially due to the extended time we are exposed to artificial lighting. This is reflected in the fact that melatonin levels of breast cancer and prostate cancer patients are half of normal.

constant exposure to artificial light has significantly reduced production of melatonin in our bodies.

- Mood Elevator
  - Nighttime melatonin levels are low in people with major depressive and panic disorders. Individuals with noticeable mood swings or who are melancholic also have depressed melatonin levels. Both seasonal affective disorder and non-seasonal cyclic depressions are related to the peaks and valleys of melatonin levels.
- Cancer Fighter
- Helps the Heart
- Relieves Asthma Symptoms
- Alzheimer's
- Cataracts
- Etc.

General Recommendations

Progesterone: Whether you're still going through your menstrual cycles (or whether you're pre-menopausal, menopausal, or post-menopausal), you need to seriously consider supplementation with an all-natural[1] progesterone cream. The benefits can be profound, and the risks of not supplementing potentially include an increased risk of breast cancer, endometrial cancer, and osteoporosis—to reiterate just a few.

- And for men, since they are not immune to the effects of xenoestrogens, low levels of natural progesterone supplementation can help with depression and can help relieve prostate problems and help prevent prostate cancer.

Estrogen: In most cases, estrogen supplementation is not called for. The problem is usually related to a lack of progesterone, not estrogen. But in those cases where it is required, make sure your doctor uses either all-natural triple-estrogen in the normal body-ratio of approximately 90% estriol, 7% estradiol, and 3% estrone—or use pure estriol. As we discussed earlier, this is the exception, not the rule; and most doctors are unaware of the difference.

Testosterone: Extracts of wild oats and nettles can safely help increase testosterone levels in the body by releasing the bound testosterone already there and

---

[1]Make sure you avoid the synthetic forms of progesterone such as Provera.

helping to prevent conversion of testosterone to dihydrotestosterone in men. For men, zinc supplementation of approximately 50 mg a day is also advisable to help prevent production of dihydrotestosterone in the body.

HGH: Supplementation with a secretagogue, a homeopathic HGH formula, or the new sublingual polymer matrix HGH makes sense for anyone over 35. All of these are okay to use on a daily basis as they do not suppress the body's own production of HGH. Of the three, however, the polymer matrix HGH is the most effective. You also might want to try increasing your exercise levels. Aerobic exercise can double HGH levels in the body, but weight training can increase levels by as much as 400–800%.

DHEA: I do not recommend supplementation with DHEA at this time without monitoring DHEA levels in your blood. If you insist, try the new 7-Keto formulas. In any case, supplementation with pregnenolone and/or HGH will help raise DHEA levels in the body. If you choose to supplement, do not use daily, as supplementation may suppress the body's own production of DHEA.

Pregnenolone: Start with 5 mg a day and increase by 5 mg a day (to a maximum of 30 mg) until you "feel" really good. Then try backing it down to the lowest level that still produces that same feeling. Finally, start backing off on the days that you use it until you are using it only 2 or 3 times a week (so as not to suppress your body's own production). As needed, as you age, you can increase the days and dosage. The final recommended dosage is age dependent. If you're younger than 50, you might consider dosages in the range of 10–20 mg 2 to 3 times a week. If you're over 50, you may end up using 15–30 mg daily.

Melatonin: Melatonin, in small doses,[1] several times a week (so as not to suppress your body's own production), makes sense for supplementation. There's virtually no downside; it can help restore optimum sleep patterns, and it's a powerful antioxidant and immune enhancer. As you get older, you can increase the amount and frequency as needed. There is, of course, another option. Use black-out curtains in the bedroom, and turn off any nightlights. Try to get the bedroom as close to total darkness as you can get. This will help increase your bodies own melatonin production. And when you wake up in the morning, expose yourself to sunlight ASAP to cut melatonin production and wake yourself up.

---

[1]Dosage varies according to what your body needs. It can range from .2 mg to 20 mg a day. The key to determining the correct dosage is that which helps you sleep, but let's you wake up without feeling "drugged." Start with .5 mg and increase by .5 mg a night until you find what works for you. Note: the effect of supplementation often carries over several nights so that you may only need to supplement every other night or every third night.

Cautions

There are several cautions that should be observed when supplementing hormones.

- Pregnant or nursing mothers should not supplement without guidance from their doctors
- Likewise, women trying to conceive would be advised to check with their doctor first
- Anyone being treated by a doctor for a pre-existing condition should check with their doctor. This would include conditions such as:
  - Autoimmune diseases
  - Cancer
  - Mental illness or depression
- Anyone on prescription steroids should check with their doctor first

In fact, it probably makes sense to check with an anti-aging specialist[1] before starting a program of hormone supplementation. Yes, that's right. There is now such a thing as an anti-aging specialist.

---

[1]Keep in mind that these specialists are still medical doctors and still prone to some of the same paradigm blindness that afflicts most doctors. Many of these specialists will recommend horse urine and synthetic progestin for women. You were given a brain. Use it, even when talking to a specialist.

CHAPTER 11

DYING OF THIRST

Clean water for drinking, bathing, and growing food is one of the most precious commodities on the planet. You constantly read in the news about how we're running out of oil and energy—how these resources can only last another 20–30 years. But the simple fact is, that's 20–30 years longer than we have for water. Already, in many parts of the world, lack of clean water is the biggest problem facing huge numbers of people.[1] Just to hazard a guess, in the next 50 years, more wars will be fought over water than oil.

Why is water so important? Quite simply, it's essential for life. And the sad fact is...most people just don't get enough. The vast majority of people living in the industrial world (even where water is abundant) are dehydrated.

QUANTITY

In advanced societies, thinking that tea, coffee, alcohol, soda pop, or other forms of manufactured beverages are desirable substitutes for the purely natural water needs of the daily "stressed" body is a common, but potentially deadly, mistake.[2]

Water is **the** solvent in our bodies, and as such, it regulates all the functions of our bodies, including the action of all the solids dissolved in the water. In fact, every function of the body is monitored and pegged to the efficient flow of water. Think for a moment of just a few of the functions that water regulates in our bodies:

- The movement of blood
- The transport of nutrients into our cells
- The movement of waste out of our cells
- The flow of lymph fluid
- The movement of nerve impulses through our nerves
- The movement of hormones throughout our bodies
- The functioning of our brains

---

[1]China is currently running a water deficit equivalent to seven times the water usage of the entire state of California. In the next few years, that deficit will **triple.** Already, the Yellow River, one of the most important rivers in China, is so low in water that it failed to reach the ocean on 226 days in 1997.

[2]Batmanghelidj, F., *Your Body's Many Cries for Water,* Falls Church: Global Health Solutions, Inc., 1995.

If we were to become dehydrated, all of these functions (and a thousand more) would be impaired. Unfortunately, that's exactly what happens for the vast majority of us. Over time, as we become increasingly dehydrated, our thirst mechanism gradually fails,[1] which leads to even more dehydration. Symptoms of chronic dehydration include allergies, asthma, chronic pains, constipation, acidosis, dry skin, and the shrinking of internal organs and thinning of skin associated with aging—to name just a few.

We need to consume between 64 and 96 ounces of pure water a day. Pure, fresh (not bottled or canned) fruit and vegetable juices may be substituted for some of this quantity—as may limited quantities of nondiuretic herbal teas (without sugar). In general, however, pure water is the key.

QUALITY

When you look at the big picture, state and federal authorities have done a remarkable job in providing "clean" water for the country as a whole. Waterborne epidemics such as cholera are almost unheard of in the United States. On the other hand, acknowledging what has been accomplished does not mean that we should close our eyes to the problems that exist.

Keep in mind that the MCLs (maximum contamination levels) that water districts so proudly adhere to merely represent a compromise standard designed to be economically feasible for water districts to meet. They in no way come close to the safety standards established by the US government's *Safe Water Drinking Act.*

On average, drinking water in the United States currently contains over 2,100 toxic chemicals that are known to cause cancer, cell mutation, and nervous disorders. This is not particularly surprising considering that there are close to 100,000 chemicals now in everyday use—with over 1,000 new ones being added each year. In fact, according to the EPA, US industries generate some 79 million pounds of toxic waste each year that is **not** disposed of properly.

What is probably more surprising to most people, though, is the fact that, according to the EPA, 53 million Americans unknowingly drink tap water that is polluted by feces, radiation, or other contaminants. Also according to the EPA, some 45 million people drink water contaminated with the parasite cryptosporidium that killed more than 100 people in Milwaukee in 1993. Or that over half of all Americans drink water that has been **used at least once before.**[2]

According to an ABC News Special, US industries generate some 88 million pounds of toxic waste a year, 90% of which the EPA estimates is improperly disposed of, which makes its way into our water supplies. With close to 100,000

[1]Even when our thirst mechanism is functioning properly, it's not a reliable indicator of dehydration since "thirst" is one of the last symptoms of dehydration to manifest.

[2]You probably shouldn't think about this particular statistic too long if you have any tendency toward a weak stomach.

chemicals now in use and with the introduction of 1,000 new ones each year, it's impossible for treatment plants to keep up. Each year, at least 400,000 cases of illness can be attributed to contaminated water.

With all due respect for the great job that all of the water departments in all of the states and cities do, you still don't want to be drinking tap water. It may not kill you immediately, but as sure as the sun rises in the morning, it will compromise your health over time. The bottom line is that you need to drink filtered (or distilled water). Tap water, well water, and bottled water[1] are all suspect.

Chlorine

Chlorine is the primary disinfectant used to purify drinking water. Let me make it absolutely clear that I am not advocating eliminating chlorine from the purification process. That would be stupid. Chlorination controls many water-borne diseases, including typhoid fever, cholera, and dysentery. When chlorination was stopped in Peru, for instance, there was a cholera epidemic of 300,000 cases.

However, it should be understood that:

- Chlorine is one of the most toxic substances known. It does everything from drying your skin and destroying your hair to wiping out the beneficial bacteria in your colon.
- And the byproducts of chlorination (such as chloroform, dichloro acetic acid, and MX), which are found in drinking water, are all proven carcinogens.
- According to the US Council on Environmental Quality, the cancer risk among people drinking chlorinated water is 93% higher than among those whose water does not contain chlorine. There is a higher incidence of cancer of the esophagus, rectum, breast, and larynx and a higher incidence of Hodgkin's disease among those drinking chlorinated water.
- Chlorine has been strongly implicated as a major factor in the onset of atherosclerosis and its resulting heart attacks and strokes.
- By the same mechanisms that chlorine narrows blood vessels that feed the heart, it also narrows the blood vessels that feed the brain. Consequently, chlorine has been implicated as a major factor in the onset of senility.

There's no question but that the use of chlorine in drinking water has helped stop the spread of many virulent water-borne diseases. On the other hand, there's also no question but that chlorine in our drinking water presents us with serious long-term health implications. **The bottom line on chlorine is that it pretty much needs to remain part of the city water purification process. That means that you need to remove it from your water at your house.**

---

[2]Yes, if you're on the road and you're thirsty, picking up some bottled water at a 7-11 is a better alternative than drinking from the water fountain or buying some coffee or soda.

Fluoride

At the risk of being accused of being a Luddite, let's take a look at the use of fluoride in our drinking water.

Exactly what is water fluoridation? In fact, all water contains some fluoride. Fluoridation is the process of adjusting the level of fluoride in the water supply to theoretically protect against tooth decay. This concentration varies from 0.7 to 1.2 parts per million (ppm). While it is true that "organic" fluoride itself is present naturally in soil, water, plants and many foods,[1] the "industrial" fluoride used in water fluoridation is a toxic waste product.[2]

Does it work? Now that's a question of more than some debate. There's no question that since fluoridation began, the incidence of dental caries has gone down significantly in the United States. Score one for water fluoridation! But hold on a second. It's gone down throughout the country—even in states that don't fluoridate their water! In fact, there is no good statistical evidence that fluoride (either in your water or your toothpaste) makes one iota of difference in terms of dental health.[3] All of the improvement in dental health that we have seen in the United States can easily be attributed to better dental hygiene (brushing and flossing), not fluoridation.Which brings us to the key question: Is it safe?

Well, to be fair, community water fluoridation is supported by the U.S. Public Health Service,[4] the American Dental Association,[5] the American Medical Association,[6] the American Heart Association, the American Cancer Society, and the National Academy of Sciences. On the other hand, the devastating, toxic effects of fluoride are well documented by mainstream organization such as:

- Numerous articles have appeared in the *New England Journal of Medicine* and the *Journal of the American Medical Association* challenging the safety of fluoridation

---

[1]Tea, for example, is an extremly high source of fluoride (even when made with unfluoridated water).

[2]American industry loves water fluoridation. Instead of having to pay for the disposal of a toxic waste product, they now **get paid** by cities by selling them this same toxic waste. It's probably no surprise then that the industries producing fluoride byproducts are some of the biggest proponents (and backers) of water fluoridation.

[3]In fact, as New Zealand's former chief dental-health officer, Jon Colquhon, a one-time proponent of fluoridation, said, "When any unfluoridated area is compared with a fluoridated area with a similar income level, the percentage of children who are free of dental decay is consistently higher in the unfluoridated area."

[4]While at the same time, curiously, pushing for a reduction in our daily fluoride intake. Maybe you can explain that to me.

[5]It's worth noting that the American Dental Association is on the horns of a dilemma. To admit that promoting the use of fluoride was a mistake would open up the floodgates of litigation.

[6]While at the same time repeatedly publishing articles in their magazine proving the dangers of fluoride. No one ever said this has to make sense.

- National Institute of Environmental and Health Sciences has shown that fluoride causes cancer.
- Scientists at the Environmental Protection Agency have come out against fluoridation because they have confirmed that it does not reduce tooth decay and that there is clear evidence that fluoride causes cancer.
- The Pasteur Institute in France, and the Nobel Institute in Sweden have caused fluoride to be banned in France and Sweden respectively because the health risks from using fluoride far outway any possible benefit.
- Fluoridation is also banned in Finland, Holland, Chile, and Japan among others.

Fluoride is a potent toxin[1] that accumulates (about 50% a day for adults and 75% a day for children) in the body. Each exposure stays in your body and adds to the accumulated levels. And that's the key. We are constantly being exposed to high levels of fluoride other than in our water. It is in our toothpaste.[2] It is sprayed on our food.[3] It is present in pharmaceutical drugs ranging from birth control pills to antibiotics. It is in soda pop, which is manufactured from fluoridated water. Once you look at the scope of the problem, you realize that there is no way in the world to determine what your flouride intake is, but it's far higher than is healthy. Health problems associated with fluoride include:

- Destruction of the immune system
- Up to a 39% increase in various cancers—with an astounding 80% increase in rectal cancer
- Genetic changes both in sperm and other cells
- Dramatic increase in heart-related deaths
- Brittle bones[4]
- Chronic fatigue

[1]Fluoride is used as a pesticide particularly for roaches, ants, and rats.

[2]Note: fluoride toothpaste can double the level of fluoride in the blood within five minutes of being used—just from the amount absorbed through the cheeks and gums.

[3]Apples and grapes are particularly high in fluoride for this reason.

[4]One of the claims for fluoride is that it helps builds bones. That claim is so deliberately misrepresentative of the truth that it borders on the criminal. Yes, while it is true that there are studies that confirm that fluoride builds **thicker** bones, it is gross misrepresentation to cite those studies without also mentioning that fluoride makes bones more brittle. And, in fact, there are numerous studies that have appeared in the *Journal of the American Medical Association* that show a significant increase in hip fractures in areas with fluoridated water. In addition, The *New England Journal of Medicine* reported that fluoride treatment of osteoporosis patients resulted in higher hip fracture rates.

- Gastrointestinal disturbances
- Increase in infant mortality
- Skin rashes after bathing
- Miscarriages
- Dizziness
- Vision problems—including blindness
- Not to mention mottled teeth

Also, it is well established that fluoride is an extremely potent enzyme inhibitor.

The bottom line is what freakin right does anyone have to force such a potentially toxic substance into your drinking water[1] **for no proven benefit.**[2]

Oh yes, I almost forgot, the aluminum/fluoride connection. New research has revealed that fluoride in drinking water makes the aluminum that we ingest more bioavailable. In the presence of fluoride, more aluminum crosses the blood-brain barrier and is deposited in the brain. As was reported in *Brain Research,* Vol. 7 84:98, the combination of aluminum and fluoride causes the same pathological changes in brain tissue that are found in Alzheimer's patients. Now don't misunderstand, I'm not saying that aluminum/fluoride is **the** cause of Alzheimer's. That would be premature. All I'm saying is that it might be prudent to limit your exposure until we know more one way or the other. Remember, even O.J. was found innocent in the end.

Bathing

As it turns out, it's not enough just to worry about the water you drink. The water you bathe and shower with is equally, if not more, important.

- You absorb more chlorine through your skin in a 15 minute hot shower[3] than you do by drinking eight glasses of that same water throughout the day. (So much for drinking bottled water.)
  - Just for fun, stop by your local swimming pool supply store and pick up a chlorine test kit. Fill a glass with some of your local tap water and test it with your kit. The water will change color according to how much chlorine there is in the water. Now fill up another glass with water from the tap. This time, soak your hand in the water for 60 seconds before testing. Notice how the water shows no chlorine. In just 60 seconds you absorbed all of the chlorine in the water into your body through your hand. The

[1]At least with toothpaste, you have a choice to buy a nonfluoride brand

[2]There are now at least 10 studies that prove as fluoride intake goes up, so does your tooth decay!

[3]Actually, when you shower, you absorb more chlorine through your lungs in the form of vapor (produced by the small droplets of hot water) than you do even through your skin.

> absorption factor is that dramatic. (The younger you are, the more absorbent your skin tends to be. And women should take special note; breast tissue is the most absorbent tissue in the body. Soak your breast in the same water, and it will clean out all of the chlorine in just 20 seconds.)

The trick is, if you want to protect your skin (and your body as well), you've got to mount a defense at the surface of the epidermis. Once a substance gets past this tough outer layer of dead skin cells, it generally has a much easier time passing through the living area of the epidermis and then into the body.

Bioavailability

Although all water consists of the same basic H20 molecules, water nevertheless varies according to how these molecules bond together to form "water molecule groups." To put it simply, it is in the size of these groupings that water differs. The smaller the groupings, the more bioavailable the water is—the more easily it is able to pass through cell walls, to circulate through your body as a whole.

What holds water molecules together in clusters is surface tension. This is what you see when you wash your car and the water beads up in droplets on the hood. When washing your car, you use detergent to break that surface tension—which makes the water wetter and better able to clean. Obviously, you can't use detergent to "improve" the bioavailability of your drinking water.

But you can use magnetics. Magnetizing your drinking water breaks its surface tension, making it wetter and more useable by your body. In addition, there's a strong secondary benefit. Applying a magnetic field to water **raises its** pH. This is of vital importance as we will see chapter 13.

General Recommendations

- You need to treat the water that comes into your house to remove the chlorine, fluoride, chemical residues, heavy metals, bacteria, parasites, etc. in your water. And you need to remove all of these toxins not only at the tap where you drink, but also where you bathe and shower. So how do you do it? You really only have four choices.

1. Get a system for the entire house that treats the water where it enters your house. This is obviously the most expensive way to answer the problem, but if you actually get a good system that removes all of the toxins, it's the best way to go.
2. There's no question that a good water distiller will provide the "cleanest" water you can get, but you need to be sure it incorporates a charcoal filter, since toxins like chlorine vaporize and recondense along with the water you're trying to clean.

- •• There's one other question to consider. Distilled water, by definition, has no mineral content. For years there has been much debate as to whether that's good or bad. "Distillerites" claim that demineralized water is more natural—like rain water and glacier water—and that minerals in the water end up in your joints. The argument against distillers is that most animals drink water that has had contact with the ground and acquired a high mineral content. Prime examples are the high mineral water of the Hunzas and the coral calcium water of the islands off of Okinawa—two areas renowned for the age and health of their inhabitants. As for me, I don't think it matters, **provided** that if you drink distilled water, you make sure that your diet and supplements provide an abundant supply of minerals.[1] And as for the question of mineral-laden water leading to joint deposits, **studies have proven that the calcium which deposits in joints comes from inside the body—leached from your own bones because of too much acid in your diet.**

3. Reverse osmosis units produce a good quality drinking water. The problem I have with them is that they waste a huge amount of water—many gallons of waste for each gallon of usable water. I'm not really sure that's justifiable nowadays with the looming water shortage we face.
4. A good water filter is your best bet, but keep in mind that a good filter will cost more than $29.95 or even $100. To find one that will truly clean your water and remove parasites, you will need to pay $250–$300.

- Drink 8-12 glasses of pure water a day.
- When possible, use glass to hold your water, not plastic. Absolutely avoid drinking water that has a strong plastic smell or taste.
- Apply a magnetic field to your water for at least 20 minutes (depending on how large your bottle is).
- If you're not using a central home purification system, remember to get a good shower filter to remove the chlorine from the water you shower in. Understand that the filter is on the shower, not the bath. The bath water (unless you fill the tub from the shower) will still be toxic.

[1]Understand, because it is devoid of minerals, distilled water is bioelectrically dead.

CHAPTER 12

YOUR MOUTH IS KILLING YOU

ALUMINUM COOKWARE

It has been known for some 20 years that aluminum, once it enters our bodies, has the tendency to accumulate in our brains, where it kills off neurons—leading to memory loss. And thanks to the significant amounts of aluminum found in food emulsifiers, antiperspirant deodorants, hair sprays, baking powder, many toothpastes, much of our drinking water, and most of our cookware, we are exposed to quite a lot of aluminum over the course of our lives. There has been much speculation, therefore, that aluminum may be one of the prime factors in the onset of Alzheimer's disease. The connection between aluminum and Alzheimer's disease became even stronger, when in 1995, Neurotoxicology reported that the widespread use of aluminum salts to purify water could account for the large numbers of people suffering from Alzheimer's.

And now, the final piece of the puzzle may have just fallen into place: the connection between aluminum and fluoride.

GIFTS FROM YOUR DENTIST

Dentists have accomplished many great things in this country in terms of promoting oral health, but on three key issues, they stand on the wrong side of history and health.

1. Fluoride
2. Mercury fillings
3. Root canals

1. Fluoride

In Chapter 11, Dying of Thirst, I discussed in some detail the evidence that fluoride is a dangerous toxic substance that has no business being added to our drinking water. But it is worth repeating here that new research has revealed that fluoride in drinking water makes the aluminum that we ingest more bioavailable.

In the presence of fluoride, more aluminum crosses the bloodbrain barrier and is deposited in the brain. As was reported in *Brain Research,* Vol. 7 84:98, the bottom line is that the combination of aluminum and fluoride causes the same pathological changes in brain tissue that are found in Alzheimer's patients.

2. Mercury fillings

The American Dental Association has resolutely maintained for years that "when mercury is combined with the metals used in dental amalgam, it's toxic properties are made harmless." If this were true, it would be miraculously fortuitous.

Amalgam, which consists of mercury, silver, tin, copper, and a trace amount of zinc, has been used by dentists for well over several hundred years—as far back, actually, as the 7th century in China. Here in the United States, mercury-based fillings made their appearance in the early 1800s.

From the beginning, there were a number of dentists who were concerned by the presence of mercury, since by that time it was fairly well known that mercury was poisonous. In fact, these concerns were so strong, that by the mid-1940s, several dental societies, including the American Society of Dental Surgeons, had joined together to stop the use of amalgam fillings. But amalgam was just too easy to work with, and whatever ill effects people experienced were too far down the road to matter, and so, in 1859, the American Dental Association was founded—primarily to promote the use of mercury amalgam as a safe and desirable tooth filling material. There were no tests done. No studies. Nothing. Amalgam was promoted because it was easy to work with. The reason the mercury was used in it was because mercury serves to "dissolve" the other-metals and make an homogenous whole.

It would be miraculous indeed if you could use one of the most toxic substances known to man with no ill effect. How was it defended? Well, the early position was that the mercury reacts with the other metals to form "a biologically inactive substance" so that none of it ever makes its way into your body. That too would have been miraculous indeed if that were true—but, of course, it is not. Numerous studies conducted in the 1970s and 80s have proven conclusively that the mercury from fillings (primarily from mercury vapor created when we chew) makes its way into the body, ending up in our lungs, heart, stomach, kidneys,[1] endocrine glands, gastrointestinal tract, jaw tissue, and our brains.[2]

Once it became irrefutable that mercury from the fillings was ending up in our bodies,[3] it then became mandatory that the ADA find a new defense. Again,

---

[1]Studies have shown that within 30 days of receiving amalgam fillings, kidney function is reduced some 50%.

[2]In effect, the denser the tissue, the greater the concentration of mercury.

[3]There have been something over 12,000 papers published to date elucidating the dangers of amalgam fillings, but the most compelling detailed the use of radioactively tagged amalgam fillings in a controlled experiment. In less than 30 days, substantial levels of the tagged mercury was found throughout the body and brain and especially in the liver and kidneys.

not based on study, but rather on convenience, it became the position of the ADA that: Well yes, maybe some mercury does make its way into the body, but at levels that are so low it has no effect on our health. And once again, it would be miraculous indeed if that were true. Unfortunately, it is not. Like so many other toxic substances, the real problem with mercury is that it is a cumulative poison. The body holds onto a significant percentage of the mercury that enters it.

Mercury is one of the most toxic metals known—more toxic even than lead. And while there is no conclusive evidence that the mercury from fillings causes any particular health problems, there are, on the other hand, a number of studies that "imply" such a relationship. First of all, there is strong evidence that mercury lowers T-Cell counts.[1] This, alone, implicates amalgam fillings in cancer,[2] autoimmune diseases, allergies, candida overgrowth, and multiple sclerosis.[3] It has also been shown that mercury interferes with the ability of the blood to carry oxygen—actually cutting its oxygen carrying capabilities by half. This would account for many instances of chronic fatigue. Mercury also has an affinity for our brains and is implicated in brain tumors and dementia.[4] And, finally, mercury has an affinity for fetal tissue—reaching higher levels in the fetus than in the mother herself—which accounts for mercury's implication in birth defects.

What about other sources of mercury entering the body? Well, seafood is of course a source. And some of the foods we eat are too. But, when all is said and done, the amount of mercury entering our bodies from amalgam fillings represents anywhere from 50–90% of the total amount.[5]

So why in the world does the ADA continue to support the use of amalgam fillings? One simple answer is: if you're in for an inch, you're in for a mile. What would the legal ramifications be if the ADA suddenly announced that they, and all the dentists connected with them, had been wrong for well over 100 years and had been slowly poisoning all Americans? Can you spell tobacco?

3. Root canals

If a tooth's pulp, which contains nerves and blood vessels becomes infected or damaged because of decay or injury, your options are often limited. Effectively, your dentist will offer you two options. You can either have the tooth pulled or the nerve removed—better known as a "root canal treatment." A root canal consists of removing the infected or diseased pulp from the tooth and sterilizing and

---

[1]A number of studies have shown removing amalgam fillings can cause T-Cell counts to rise anywhere from 50–300%.

[2]In fact, there have been several studies that have shown that white blood-cell abnormalities, such as found in leukemia, tend to normal out when amalgam fillings are removed.

[3]Mercury levels in MS patients is, on average, 7.5 times higher than normal.

[4]The famous mad hatters of England were the hat makers who worked with mercury and eventually went mad.

[5]Every single amalgam filling in your mouth pumps, on average, some 3,000,000,000,000,000 mercury atoms into your body each and every day.

refilling the canals with a sealer[1] to prevent recontamination of the root canal system.

In order to understand the problem, you need to first understand that a tooth is not a solid inanimate structure. Each single tooth is a living structure sustained by some 3 miles of microscopic tubules running through the solid dentin. In a healthy tooth, those tubules, which make up a full 90% of the actual tooth, can be thought of as the tooth's "arteries and veins."

Once a tooth has had it's root filled, it no longer has any nourishment circulating through it's tubules, but the tubules themselves remain—unfilled. And therein lies the problem. It is physically impossible to fully sterilize the miles of microscopic tubules in a tooth. Some bacteria survive[2] and thrive in these empty tubules. And once sealed in your tooth, no part of your immune system can reach those bacteria and destroy them, because you have sealed off the root of the tooth stopping all blood supply to the tooth's interior. And for the same reason, no antibiotics that you might take can reach the bacteria. Nevertheless, because the tooth itself is porous, those bacteria, and/or their toxins, can migrate out into surrounding tissue where they can "hitch hike" to other locations in the body via the bloodstream. The new location can be any organ or gland or tissue, and the new colony will be the next focus of infection in a body plagued by recurrent or chronic infections.

Understand, every single root canal leaks—without exception. Bacteria and/or toxins leach out from every root canal–treated tooth. Every single person who has had a root canal has had their immune system compromised by having to fight a continual low-grade infection **that it can never fully eliminate**, because it can never reach the source of that infection in the tooth itself. About 25% of all people seem to have immune systems that are strong enough to resist the continual infection coming from the tooth, thereby preventing it from taking hold anywhere else in the body for many years. But as for the other 75% . . . they can look forward to a whole range of chronic and debilitating diseases, including:

- Arthritis
- Heart disease
- Chronic infection
- Chronic fatigue
- Eye problems
- etc.

---

[1]The traditional sealer of choice in this country has been gutta percha, although new options are becoming available that overcome the major problem associated with gutta percha (microscopic shrinkage as it dries, leaving empty space in the root, which bacteria love to fill). Nevertheless, the one problem that no sealer can overcome is that no filling can reach into the miles of tubules in the tooth.

[2]Including strains of streptococcus, staphylococcus and spirochetes.

The bottom line is that root canals, at this point in time, are to be avoided. Also, for what it's worth, with better dental care and by following the dietary principles outlined in this book, you should never have to face the need for a root canal. Incidentally, if you already have a root canal and need to have it removed, it is not enough to simply have it pulled. It is almost a surety that the bacteria have migrated to the bone and tissues adjacent to the tooth's root. You will need to find a dentist experienced in the procedure for removing a root canal tooth, which includes removing the periodontal ligament (which is always infected with toxins produced by streptococcus bacteria living in the dentin tubules) and the first millimeter of bone that lines the socket (which is also usually infected).

General Recommendations

- **Aluminum.** Make sure it's not in the water you drink, and you might want to think twice about the antiperspirant you use. And finally, you might want to think about stainless steel cookware. It's okay to use cookware that has an aluminum core, as long as the food never touches the aluminum itself.
- **Fluoride.** If there's any way to keep it out of your city water supply, fight to do that. If it's already there, you have to make sure you remove it at your house so that it doesn't make it into your drinking water, bath, or shower. Also, you'll probably want to avoid fluoride toothpastes, and you'll definitely want to avoid fluoride "treatments" from your dentist.
- **Mercury fillings.** Unless you have some chronic health condition, you may not want to go through the expense of having your fillings replaced.[1] However, you would be well advised to go on some of the cleansing programs we have described earlier—particularly the colon cleanse and some form of blood cleansing, such as chelation therapy (or the use of cilantro pesto and malic acid). And if you need any new fillings, don't.
- **Root canals.** Don't. And if you have one, you may want to consider having it pulled.

---

[1]And if you are going to have your fillings removed, go to a dentist who specializes in the removal of amalgam fillings. There's a whole procedure involved so that you don't end up getting huge amounts of powdered mercury down your throat and clouds of mercury vapor up into your nasal passages as a result of the high-speed drill used to remove the amalgam.

CHAPTER 13

CLEANSING YOUR LIVER AND BLOOD

DETOXIFYING YOUR LIVER

Our liver is the primary filter of our body. Good health is impossible without proper function of the liver. Unfortunately, over time, we so abuse it and so overtax it that illness is the inevitable result. As part of a program to rebuild and repair the liver, we must:

- Remove all the excess fat from the liver.
- Get bile flowing freely again.
- Eliminate toxic waste that our livers have filtered out.
- Dissolve and pass out the accumulated gall stones that are stored in our livers.
- Regenerate the damaged and destroyed cells of the liver.

Next to the skin, the liver is the largest organ in the body. In many ways, it is the most important organ in the body, and the last to be considered when it comes to health. In addition to being large, the liver is also a complicated organ involved in at least 200 separate functions. Generally speaking, the liver performs a vital role in regulating, synthesizing, storing, secreting, transforming, and breaking down many different substances in the body. Specifically, some of these include:

- Regulation of fat stores
- Cleansing the blood and discharging waste products
- Neutralizing and destroying poisons
- Protein metabolism, including manufacturing of new body proteins
- Metabolizing alcohol
- Managing chemicals and drugs in the blood
- Aiding the digestive process by the production of bile

- Helping the body resist infections by producing immune factors and by removing bacteria from the blood stream
- Storing vitamins, minerals, and sugars
- Production of quick energy when needed
- Controlling the production and excretion of cholesterol
- Maintaining hormone balance
- Regenerating its own damaged tissue

The liver is so important to our well-being that many healers maintain that most diseases cannot develop in the body (that, in fact, no form of cell degeneration can occur) if the liver is functioning in an efficient, healthy manner. Conversely, an unhealthy liver is very likely at the root of most serious health problems.

So What Harms the Liver?

- **Too much protein in the diet.** Protein metabolism is especially taxing on the liver since it is the liver which must metabolize complex proteins into simple compounds. The greater the consumption of protein, the greater the stress on the liver.
- **Too many simple carbohydrates in the diet.** The body converts excess simple carbohydrates into triglycerides, which are then stored in the liver as fat. The more fat stored in the liver, the harder it is for the liver to perform its full range of normal functions.
- **Overeating.** Too much enzyme deficient food stresses the liver.
- **Drug residues.** Virtually all of the drugs that we take (medicinal, recreational, chemotherapy, whatever) are processed, purified, and refined in the liver—in preparation for elimination from the body.
- **Alcohol causes inflammation of the liver's tissue.** Once the liver is inflamed, it can no longer filter, which causes it to plug up with fat and become even more inflamed. If we consume enough alcohol, we overwhelm the liver's ability to regenerate itself, and the net result is cirrhosis (or hardening) of the liver.
- **Toxins, heavy metals, and pesticides.** Everything we breathe, eat, and absorb through our skin is purified and refined in the liver.
- **Lack of exercise** forces the liver to do the elimination work that should be done by the lungs and the skin.
- **And of course, there's liver disease such as chronic Hepatitis C.**

What Are the Symptoms of Liver Dysfunction?

- Digestive problems
- Constipation
- Low energy output
- Allergies and hay fever
- Arthritis
- Diabetes
- Hypertension
- Obesity
- Infertility

So What Can Be Done About It?

Fortunately, your liver has an astounding ability to regenerate itself—if you give it a chance. Giving it a chance means two things:

- **The Don'ts**
  - In Chapter 6, we discussed the elements of proper diet. Well, they particularly apply in terms of the liver. You need to eliminate (or at least cut back) the liver stressors in your diet. The sicker you are, the more cleaned up your diet needs to be. If you're suffering from serious liver problems, a raw juice diet may be required to give your liver time to regenerate.
- **The Do's**
  - Several times a year, you need to do an herbal detox/flush of your liver. A low level cleanse using betaine hydrochloride and pancreatic enzymes is also helpful.
  - You need to regularly include nutritional support for the liver. Look for formulas that contain milk thistle, dandelion root, the perennial herb Picrorhiza kurooa,[1] and artichoke or beet leaf.

And Finally, a Word About the Gallbladder

The poor gallbladder. Guilty by being found at the scene of the crime, it is the frequent target of the surgeon's knife. Gallbladder removal is one of the most frequently performed operations in America.[2]

---

[1]Picrorhiza has been shown to protect liver cells from the many degenerative changes that would normally be caused by a variety of liver toxins. It appears to be particularly useful in treating both alcoholic liver damage and chronic viral hepatitis.

[2]Over a half-million gallbladders are removed each year in the United States.

Understand, the gallbladder is not responsible for the production of gallstones. The liver is the culprit—or rather what we do to the liver. The gallbladder is merely a holding area for bile to be used in the digestion of fats and oils. But if our diets are too high in the wrong kind of oils, if we have allergies to dairy and eggs, low levels of stomach acid, too little fiber in our diets, stress, if the liver is not functioning properly, etc., etc., etc., why then the bile produced in the liver (a mixture of cholesterol, minerals, bile salts, pigment, and lecithin) is of a type and consistency that tends to quickly harden into "stones" before it can be passed out of the gallbladder.[1]

Removing the gallbladder does not remove the problem; it merely removes the symptoms. Yes, it's true that after gallbladder removal you're unlikely to suffer from further gallstones. But on the other hand, you've now traded one problem for two new ones:

1. Since you never corrected the underlying problem of imbalances in the liver, these problems will just continue to get worse—eventually compromising the liver itself.

2. By removing the gallbladder, you also remove its regulating effect on bile. That means that bile is continually dumping into your intestinal tract when it is not needed, and is available in only minimal amounts when it is needed. The net result is chronic digestive problems and probable long-term nutritional deficiencies.

Far better than removing the gallbladder is a seasonal liver/gallbladder flush combined with a periodic liver rebuilding program.

Liver/Gallbladder Flush

By cleansing the liver, we're talking about inducing the liver to purge all of the fats, old cholesterol deposits, gallstones, poisons, drug residues, and toxic waste stored therein. Probably nothing else you do (including even the bowel cleanse and detox) will make a greater difference in your overall health.

Note: It is vital that you do a colon cleanse before doing the liver cleanse. When the liver dumps, it dumps through the bile duct and out into the colon. If the colon (the drain pipe if you will) is plugged, the waste backs up into the blood stream and can make you feel extremely ill. This is the reason that the miracle doctors always start with the colon detox. It's the prerequisite for all the other cleanses in the body—and, of course, can also produce dramatic healings in its own right.

The 5-Day Cleanse

This is the Liver/Gallbladder flush recommended by Dr. Richard Schulze—and

[1]Women, incidentally, are four times more likely than men to get gallstones.

is the one most people should opt for. It is done in the morning on an empty stomach for 5 days.

First thing on rising, drink 8 ounces of pure water to flush your digestive tract.

An hour later, in a blender, mix up 8 ounces of any fresh squeezed citrus juice (fresh squeezed apple juice or grape juice with all the sediment will work too), one lemon, 1 clove of garlic (increase by 1 clove each day), 1 tablespoon of olive oil (increase by 1 tablespoon each day), and a piece of ginger (about 1-inch long) along with 8 ounces of pure water

Drink it down and follow with a fresh juice chaser to clear your mouth.

Fifteen minutes after consuming this drink, follow with 2 cups of the liver/detox tea. It is also important to take 2 droppersful of the liver/detox tincture 3–6 times a day while on the 5-day cleanse—and continuing after until the bottle is gone.

The Detox Diet

It is extremely beneficial to incorporate a 2-day raw food and 3-day juice fast into your 5-day cleanse.

- **Day 1**

  During the morning (after your cleansing drink and stopping one hour before lunch), eat all the live **fresh** fruit or vegetable juice you want. Beet juice is especially good. Do not mix your fruit and vegetable juices together, and feel free to dilute your juices.

  For lunch you can have more diluted juice, or a raw vegetable or sprout salad. Absolutely do not use bottled dressing. Make your own dressing from fresh olive oil and lemon or apple cider vinegar and any fresh herbs and spices you of your choice. If you are hungry throughout the day, feel free to snack on fresh vegetables or juices. For dinner eat fresh fruit or fruit juice or fruit smoothies.

- **Days 2–4**

  After your morning flush, drink diluted juices and herbal tea throughout the day—as much as you can drink. Try to consume 128 ounces during the day.

  Also recommended throughout the day is to consume cups of potassium broth. Potassium broth takes advantage of the fact that the outside of a potato is one of the highest plant sources of potassium. Take the peelings (¼" to ½" including the skin) of several potatoes. Do **not** use the inside. Add other well chopped vegetables to taste including carrots (with skin), celery, whole beets (including greens), fresh parsley, and lots of onion and garlic (up to 50 cloves).

  Simmer for 40–60 minutes in a covered pot using clean filtered water. Strain out the vegetables, cool and drink the broth. Refrigerate leftover broth in glass containers in the refrigerator for use over the next 2 days.

- **Day 5**

  Same as Day 1

30-Day Cleanse

Eat 1 cup of freshly grated beets mixed with olive oil and lemon for 30 days straight.

Daily use of the liver/detox tea and tincture is also required.

What Can You Expect?

If you are so inclined (and you should be) you should examine what you deposit in the toilet. Look for "stones." The bile from the liver gives some stones their pea green color. But also look for black stones and red ones and brown ones. And look for stones with blood inside them.

During the course of a cleanse, it's not uncommon to pass some 2,000 of these stones. Be glad. The more you pass, the healthier you become. You may also find untold numbers of tiny white cholesterol "crystals" mixed in with the waste.

The Liver/Detox Tea & Tincture

The use of an herbal tea and tincture along with the flush is essential.

- **The Tea**

The tea helps with the flushing process itself, but also helps minimize any discomfort or nausea. The key herb in the tea is dandelion root, one of the strongest herbal lipotropics known. That is to say, it flushes fat deposits from the liver. Other herbs that you will find in a good detox tea include things like ginger, clove, cinnamon, burdock root, and horsetail.

Incidentally, some of the other herbs used in a good liver/detox tea (such as uva ursi, parsley root, and juniper berries) are also extremely beneficial to the kidneys.

Two cups of the tea should be consumed fifteen minutes after drinking your citrus and olive flush. But several cups can and should be consumed throughout the day. In fact, consuming the liver/detox tea as a regular part of your diet is a pleasant and tasty way to continually optimize your health. (Feel free to sweeten the tea with honey or real maple syrup as desired.)

- **The Tincture**

The tincture is crucial in that it contains herbs that help the liver to rebuild and regenerate itself. A secondary benefit is that it will significantly reduce the liver's release of LDL cholesterol. The key herbs include milk thistle, dandelion root, the perennial herb picrorhiza kurooa (sometimes called kutkin, or "Indian milk thistle"), and artichoke or beet leaf.

The liver/detox tincture is also a good place to include the antiparasitic herbs such as wormwood and black walnut. Along with the garlic that you are taking with the liver flush, this will drive virtually any parasite from your body.

Take 2 droppersful 3–6 times a day (depending on your level of illness and your level of discomfort) until the entire bottle is gone.

The Blood

Our blood is filled with many impurities including everything from an overabundance of fats and cholesterol, to toxic heavy metals. These must be removed from the blood for optimum health.

The idea of blood cleansing goes back to the middle ages; and, when you think about it, the concept of "cleaning" the blood probably resonates with today's medical establishment about as well as bloodletting and philosopher's stones. Nevertheless, it works—and what's more, it even makes sense.

The concept that we eventually overwhelm our body's ability to remove all of the toxins from our blood is not really too hard to imagine, especially if we actually think about what it is we eat and drink. Does anyone really believe that the body is capable of removing the waste created in a life of eating high-fat fast-food burgers, french fries cooked in beef fat, countless large colas containing 32 teaspoons of sugar, and cream-filled donuts boiled in lard and packed with hydrogenated oil and sugar filling. Then, to top it all off at the end of the day, a half pound of beef jerky and a bag of pork rinds, accompanied by a six pack of beer just to teach the liver a lesson?

Okay, so maybe you don't do all that. But remember, what you do do, you do **day after day, year after year.** Eventually:

- Your blood can no longer remove everything you throw at it. It becomes "toxic" and thick—burbling like sludge through your arteries.
- The quality of your blood (cells and plasma) is compromised by the quality of the food you eat. Your blood totally replaces itself every 120 days. How can you possibly expect to be building high-quality blood on a diet of pepperoni pizza, beer, and twinkies?

Eventually, you need to correct the problem on multiple levels, or face long term degenerative illness.

- You have to do a general cleaning of the blood.
- You have to remove all of the heavy metals and excess cholesterol.
- You have to address the issue of blood pH.
- You have to eat the right kinds of food and supplements so that your body can begin producing, once again, healthy blood.

Cleansing the Blood

There is no secret as to which herbs cleanse the blood. Despite what medical doctors may think, the efficacy of these herbs has been proven over several hundred years. Just because medical science doesn't yet know why these herbs work as blood cleansers, doesn't mean that they don't. They do. Any good blood cleansing formula will contain some, or all, of the following herbs: Red clover blossoms, Burdock root, Chaparral, Periwinkle, and Goldenseal.[1]

The Chelators

Over 300,000 bypasses a year are now performed in US hospitals, at well over $40,000 each. It works out to something like $15 billion dollars a year spent on coronary bypasses. At least 5% of the patients die from the procedure; even more die from complications such as stroke. But what the heck, it's a small risk and a small price to pay since there's no alternative. Right?

Well, not exactly. As it turns out, there is an alternative that's so effective that in countries such as New Zealand, it's against the law to perform a bypass unless this alternative has been tried first. This therapy is called chelation treatment, and it could save hundreds of thousands of lives a year. Unfortunately, it costs just a fraction of what a coronary bypass or angioplasty costs. In other words, since chelation therapy would cost the medical establishment billions of dollars a year, it's not surprising they don't use it.

Chelation therapy has two pronounced effects on the body.

1. It chelates (or claws) onto heavy metals such as aluminum, lead, and mercury (particularly those located in the cardiovascular system) and pulls them out of your body.

2. By removing heavy metals from the body, chelation therapy significantly reduces the production of free radicals in the blood stream and the consequent scarring of the arterial walls.

The net result for most people is a dramatic improvement in the health and condition of their cardiovascular system. If you're in an advanced state of coronary disease, you should seriously consider tracking down a doctor who specializes in EDTA chelation therapy.

Note: chelation therapy is not for everyone. It involves going to a doctor's office for a series of approximately 30 four-hour intravenous "drip" sessions. In addition, although it costs a fraction of what bypass surgery costs, it is not inexpensive—usually running a little over $2,000 for the complete set of 30 sessions. On the other hand, if you are not in an "advanced state," there is an even easier alternative.

---

[1]Poke root is one of the greatest blood cleansers, but the FDA has made it difficult to find any formulas that actually incorporate poke root.

Oral Chelation

Oral chelation is not as quick as chelation therapy, Nevertheless, given a little time, it can do an extremely effective job at cleaning out the blood. Oral chelation formulas are usually based on one of two key ingredients:

- Most formulas are based on EDTA. EDTA works great when administered directly into the blood stream through standard chelation therapy, but it's usefulness when taken orally is open to question. There are some studies that indicate that there may be less than 5% absorption when taken orally.
- There's really only one oral chelator that's "proven." It's relatively expensive and difficult to handle, which is why you rarely find it (at adequate dosages) in oral chelation formulas. It's cysteine. Oral chelation formulas based on cysteine need to provide a good 750 mg of cysteine[1] in a day's dosage. The tablets also need to be protected from the air since cysteine oxidizes easily and turns black and smelly when exposed to air. Keep in mind, however, that oral chelation formulas with cysteine have a couple of problems that need to be addressed.
    - High doses of cysteine can cause kidney stones to form; therefore, the chelation formula must include adequate amounts of vitamin C (about 4,000–5,000 mgs a day) to prevent the formation of kidney stones.
    - Also, there is a risk when high levels of cysteine are used that the body will convert it to homocysteine—not good for the heart. High levels of the B vitamins (particularly folic acid), however, will prevent conversion of the cysteine to homocysteine.

Two Low-Cost Chelation Alternatives

- An interesting low-cost alternative may have recently emerged. Initial studies indicate that fresh cilantro may be extremely effective in helping flush heavy metals out of the blood. Taking 400 mg of cilantro a day can pretty much clean heavy metals out of the body in just 2–3 weeks.[2] Dr. David Williams has a great recipe for cilantro pesto in his June '98 *Alternatives* newsletter.
    - Process one cup packed **fresh** cilantro and six tablespoons of olive oil in a blender until the cilantro is chopped. Add one clove garlic; a half cup almonds, cashews, or other nuts, and two tablespoons lemon juice. Blend to a lumpy paste. (Add a little hot water if necessary.) Eat a couple of teaspoons a day for three weeks to clean out the heavy metals. Repeat 2 or 3 times a year. Be careful; it tastes incredible and is addictive. (Note: the pesto freezes nicely, so you can make several batches at once.)

---

[1]As a comparison, the yolk of one egg contains about 250 milligrams of cysteine. But in an egg the cysteine is offset by all the other essential amino acids in the egg.

[2]This can be determined by tracking the rise and fall of heavy metal levels found in the urine when fresh cilantro is consumed over a 3-week period.

- The other chelator is malic acid. Malic acid is found in fresh apples and apple cider vinegar. Malic acid is particularly useful in removing aluminum from the body.

Balancing pH

Our bodies function in a very narrow range of acid/alkaline balance (pH). Our blood in particular is very sensitive to these changes. Ideally, blood pH should be slightly alkaline at about 7.45. If it varies by even as little as a few tenths of a point, severe illness and death may result. Unfortunately, most of the food we eat is highly acidic (meat, dairy, sodas, alcohol, cooked grains). In the end, it becomes too much for our bodies to handle. If we don't correct the problem by "alkalinizing" the body, disease, sickness, and death are the inevitable result.

What is pH? It's simply the measurement of the acid/alkaline balance of anything.

- On the pH scale, water is neutral and rates a 7.0 on the scale.
- Acids (such as hydrochloric acid and citric acid) are rated as numbers less than 7.0. The further away from 7.0 the number is, the stronger the acid. Cow's milk at 6.5 is slightly acidic; Soft drinks at 3.0 are strongly acidic; and stomach acid at 1.5 is highly acidic.
- Alkaline substances include everything that rates above 7.0 on the pH scale. Again, as with acids, the further away from 7.0 the number, the more alkaline the substance. Blood at 7.45 is slightly alkaline; pancreatic juice in your intestines is strongly alkaline at 8.8, and baking soda at 12.0 is highly alkaline.

Your body has a whole bunch of different pHs that it has to maintain. Your saliva is slightly alkaline. Your stomach is strongly acidic. Your intestines are strongly alkaline. Your urine is acid. **But of all the pHs in your body, the most crucial is your blood. If your blood pH deviates even $^{5}/_{10}$ths of a point from its normal pH of 7.45, death is likely.** Considering the importance of pH to the body, it's well worth discussing a little further how it affects the body, and how we can help maintain the proper pH levels in our own bodies.

The importance of pH really boils down to two things:

1. **Enzymes.** We've already discussed the importance of enzymes. They control every single metabolic function in our bodies, and they are integral to our immune system. As it says in *Anatomy and Physiology* by Anthony and Thibodeau, **"Enzymes function optimally at a specific pH** and become inactive if this deviates beyond narrow limits."
2. **Oxygen.** Every cell in our body requires oxygen for life—and to maintain optimum health. To put it simply, the more acid the blood, the less oxygen is available for use by the cells. Without going into a discussion of the

chemistry involved, just understand that it's the same mechanism involved when acid rain "kills" a lake. The fish literally suffocate to death because the acid in the lake "binds up" all of the available oxygen. It's not that the oxygen has gone anywhere; it's just no longer available. Conversely, if you raise the pH of the lake, oxygen is now available and the lake comes back to life. Incidentally, it's worth noting that cancer is related to an acid environment (lack of oxygen). The higher the pH (the more oxygen present in the cells of the body), the harder it is for cancer to thrive.

The bottom line is that a balanced pH is vital. **An extended pH imbalance of any kind threatens our well-being—threatens, in fact, our very lives.** Managing the pH balance of all of our bodily fluids is so important that our bodies have developed systems to monitor and balance acid-alkaline levels in every cell and biosystem.

What Affects pH in Our Bodies?

As I just mentioned, our bodies have developed a system for maintaining pH balance in all of our body fluids. To understand this system better, we need to take a look at what changes pH (usually making us more acid), and how our bodies respond to that change.

- When they are metabolized, carbohydrates, proteins, and fats produce various acids in our bodies. Proteins produce sulfuric acid and phosphoric acid. Carbohydrates and fats produce acetic acid and lactic acid. Since these acids are poisonous to the body, they must be eliminated. Unfortunately, they can't be eliminated through the kidneys or large intestine as they would damage these organs.
  - **Acid-Forming Foods**

    All meats, fish, poultry, eggs, dairy, cooked grains, and refined sugars. (Note: probably at the top of the list in the human diet is soda pop. Not only is it high in refined sugar, which is highly acid forming in and of itself, but most soda pop contains a large amount of phosphoric acid—not to mention carbon dioxide (an end product of the acid neutralization process.)
  - **Alkaline-Forming Foods**

    Only fresh fruits and vegetables are alkaline-forming and help your body maintain a proper pH. (Note: even though citrus fruits are highly acidic, your body treats them as alkaline so that they are highly effective alkalinizers.)
- Since the body cannot eliminate acids through the kidneys, the way it handles them is to neutralize them with the minerals sodium, calcium, potassium, and magnesium. Of these, calcium is the most important. **Now, here's the key to the whole deal. Your body makes use of a priority system if there are not**

enough available minerals to neutralize all of the acids present.

- •• Blood is at the top of the pack. Your body will steal minerals from anywhere and everywhere before it will let your blood go too acidic. Remember, even a slight deviation in blood pH results in death.
- •• Saliva is at the bottom of the pack. Saliva is the first place your body steals minerals from to balance the blood. That's why pH testing saliva provides an early warning system for when you are becoming too acidic. At optimum health, your saliva will test at 7.45. At 6.5-7.0, you'll find yourself frequently succumbing to colds and sickness. **At 5.5 and lower, you can pretty much count on the fact that major disease has already taken hold. Virtually, all cancer patients test strongly acidic on a saliva pH test.**
- •• Unfortunately, your saliva just doesn't contain that big a reserve of minerals so you soon run out. That places your bones next on the priority list. Surprise, your bones are your body's prime mineral reserve. That's right, if your diet is too acid forming (too much meat, dairy, carbohydrates, and sugars), your body will begin leaching calcium from your bones to balance the pH and avoid death. In effect, your body says osteoporosis is preferable to death.

How Can We Help?

- Change your diet. Follow the guideline laid out in Chapter 6.
- In addition, there are several special alkalinizing agents available.
  - •• Your health food store has alkalinizing teas or drops available.
  - •• There is a machine from Japan that will "micronize" your water. What it actually does is take your tap water and divide it in two. One stream is acidic and can be used for washing and cleaning. The other steam is alkaline and is used for drinking. It works really well. Unfortunately, it's really expensive—about $1,200.
  - •• One of the best alternatives is to simply magnetize your water. Applying a magnetic field to a pitcher of water for a short period of time will make it more alkaline. It also offers the added advantage of lessening the surface tension, which makes the water wetter and more usable by the cells of your body.

General Recommendations

Liver

- **Liver/Gallbladder flush.** A liver/gallbladder flush 2–4 times a year (even more often if ill) to eliminate any accumulation of liver fat, toxins, and incipient gallstones is mandatory.

- **Liver rebuilding tonic.** In addition to flushing, you need to regularly partake of a liver rebuilding tonic. Such a tonic does three things. Herbs such as milk thistle stimulate the liver to rebuild itself. Picrorhiza kurooa serves to protect the liver. And herbs such as dandelion root, barberry, artichoke, and beet leaf are lipotropics that help to clean the fat out of the liver.
- Regular consumption of fresh apple/beet juice is profoundly beneficial to the liver.
- Note: never do a liver cleanse without first cleaning out the colon to provide an outlet for the toxins released by the liver.

Blood

- **Cleansing.** 2–4 times a year (even more often if ill) you need to go on an herbal cleansing of the blood.
- Note: never do a blood cleanse without first cleaning out the colon to provide an outlet for the toxins released by the blood.
- **Oral Chelation.** 3–4 times a year for a period of 2–3 weeks at a time, use either:
    - Cilantro pesto as described earlier in the chapter.
    - Malic acid tablets.
    - If you want, you can also use one of the low-level oral chelators on the market.
- **Alkalinize or Die.**
    - Cut way back on acid-producing foods such as meat, dairy, sugar, soda pop, refined grains, etc. Add alkalinizing foods to your diet.
    - Drink water that has been magnetized. Magnetizing can raise the pH by as much as one full point, depending on the water.
    - One final thought on pH. It really makes sense to test the pH of your saliva on a regular basis as a touchstone of your overall health. You can pick up pH paper specifically designed for this purpose at most health food stores. Make sure you test in the morning before brushing or eating as these things can temporarily alter the pH in your mouth. Just spit out a couple of times into the sink, then onto the pH paper. Ideally, your pH should be about 7.45. If it tests below 7.0, you should get aggressive in terms of alkalinizing your body.
- **Fasting.** There are any number of books on fasting to help guide you through the process. The principles of fasting are simple.
    - First, when you deprive your body of food, your body begins to consume

itself to survive. Being geared to self-survival, your body chooses to consume damaged cells and toxic cells first, saving the healthiest for later.

- It takes a tremendous amount of energy, and puts a tremendous strain on your body's organs, to process food. (Check your heart rate after eating a large meal and observe how exhausted you feel.) When you fast, your body diverts that energy to repair and rebuilding.
- No matter what medical doctors may say, the process works. In fact, a simple thought that should clue you in to the necessity for periodic fasting is the fact that **human beings are the only animals that eat when they're sick.** Think about that for a moment. Have you ever observed how dogs or cats, for example, stop eating while they're recovering? They intuitively understand the healing power of fasting. There are three levels of fasting worth considering.

1. **The pure water fast.** This is the most powerful, but also produces the most toxic side effects. I do not recommend it unless you have a great deal of experience in fasting or are working directly with a qualified healer.
2. **Juice fasting.** Fasting on fresh juices helps smooth out many of the negatives of fasting.
3. **Spirulina or Chlorella fasting.** Even gentler is supplementing your juice fast with spirulina or chlorella throughout the day.

- The one thing you need to be careful of while fasting is the build up of ketones in the body. Make sure you drink large amounts of water to flush the ketones from your body.
- One final note on fasting. In Chapter 3, we discussed the herbal colon-activator formula that provides both cleansing and healing to the entire gastrointestinal system. It's highly recommended that you use such a formula while fasting to accelerate removal of toxins from the colon. If not, you will have to take a colonic or an enema every day.

Chapter 14

Optimizing Your Immune System

Your immune system plays two vital roles in your body.

1. First, it responds to foreign organisms by producing antibodies and stimulating specialized cells which destroy those organisms or neutralize their toxic products. In this manner, it defends against foreign invaders: germs, viruses, bacteria, and the like.
2. And second, it stands guard over the cells of your body to ensure that they are not abnormal or degenerating.[1]

Your Immune System

In many ways, your immune system is the most awesome system in your body, easily rivaling your brain in terms of complexity, subtlety, and "self-awareness." Just a sample of the things your immune system does includes:

- Your immune system is capable of identifying every single cell in your body and recognizing each and every one as friendly.
- Conversely, it's capable of singling out and identifying foreign invaders ranging from bacteria and viruses to fungi and parasites.
- Once it has identified an invader, your immune system then quickly develops a customized defense weapon that specifically targets the invader's weak spot.
- Then, it gets even better. Having designed the specific weapon required, your immune system then begins building factories that produce these weapons in massive quantities sufficient to totally crush an invader.
- And once the invader has been defeated, the immune system has the awareness to "shut itself down"—to go, as they say in the military, from DEFCON 5 to DEFCON 1.

[1]Normally, there are anywhere between 100 to 10,000 abnormal cells floating around in our bodies at any point in time.

- And as amazing as all of this is, we haven't yet come to the three most amazing aspects of the immune system—the aspects that highlight its **intelligence.**
  - First, once it has defeated an invader, your immune system remembers that invader and the defense that was used to defeat it. If that invader ever makes another appearance, even decades later, your immune system can launch its defense instantly.
  - Even more amazing, however, is the fact that your immune system can identify when a cell in your body has changed, has "gone over to the enemy" as it were. This is stunning sophistication. Out of all the trillions of cells in your body, your immune system can tell when one single cell has mutated and become cancerous—and, in most cases, move in and destroy it before it can do any harm. In fact, it does this **thousands of times a day.**
  - And, then, most amazing of all, your immune system is in total communication with each and every part of itself. "So what's the big deal," you might ask? "The brain does the same thing." Yes, but remember, the billions and billions of cells of the immune system **are not in physical contact with each other.** To paraphrase Einstein, "At its core, the immune system resembles nothing so much as a **great thought.**"

In the next few paragraphs, I'm going to try and summarize the functioning of your immune system. In reality, a full discussion would take several volumes just to clarify the limited amount that we know about it at this point in time. Nevertheless, what I would like to do is at least give you a brief summary, a sense if you will, a context for how this marvelous system works.

The Parts of Your Immune System

All blood cells, both red and white, begin as stem cells in your bone marrow. These undifferentiated cells begin to assume individual characteristics and become either red cells (the oxygen carriers) or white cells (the cells of the immune system). Further differentiation divides the white cells (also called leukocytes) into four main types of cells:

1. Lymphocytes
2. Phagocytes
3. Granulocytes
4. Dendritic cells

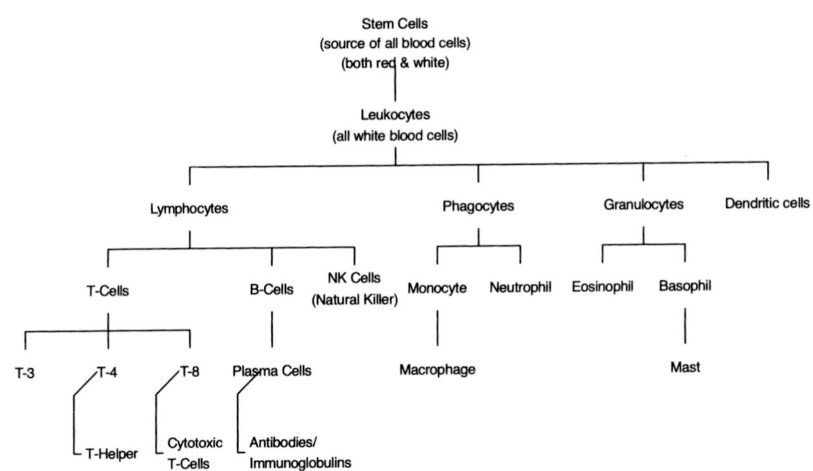

Lymphocytes

Lymphocytes are small white blood cells that serve as the key operatives of the immune system. In a healthy body, not under attack, they number about one trillion. There are three main classes of lymphocytes.

1. B-Cells. Each B-Cell is programmed to make one specific antibody[1] to defend against one specific invader. For example, one B-Cell produces an antibody to defend against only one particular strain of flu, whereas it takes an entirely different B-Cell to produce the antibody for a different strain of flu and a third B-Cell for the strep bacteria. B-Cells work primarily in the fluids of the body and work at defending against "foreign" invaders and toxic molecules. They are not capable of defending against the body's own cells that have "gone bad."

   Once a B-Cell encounters the particular invader that it is built to defend against,[2] it produces many large plasma cells. Plasma cells are nothing less than "factories" that produce millions and millions and millions of specific antibodies and release them into the blood stream. Once the invader has been eliminated, the B-Cells stop production of the plasma cells and go back to their waiting mode.

---

[1]An antibody is a soluble protein produced by B-Cells that's capable of binding to and destroying or neutralizing one specific foreign substance (also called an antigen) in the body. Antibodies belong to a particular family of nine proteins called the immunoglobulins.

[2]Although B-Cells are capable of recognizing invaders on their own, primarily that function falls to the T-Cells.

2. **T-Cells** are smarter than B-Cells. They've been to school as it were. After being produced in the bone marrow, T-Cells make their way to the Thymus where they are eductated in how to distinguish between the cells of the body and invading cells—and to distinguish between normal healthy cells and mutated rogue cells.[1] Every T-Cell carries a marker, a distinctive molecule on its surface, that effects how it behaves. Every T-Cell carries a T-3 marker.
   - In addition, some T-Cells carry a T-4 marker. These are known as the T-Helper Cells, which serve the purpose of identifying foreign invaders—then activating B-Cells, other T-Cells, Natural Killer Cells, and Macrophages to attack the invader.
   - And finally, some T-Cells carry a T-8 marker. Most T-8 Cells are known as Cytotoxic T-Cells,[2] which identify rogue mutated cells in the body or cells that have been invaded by viruses and compromised. Once they've identified the enemy, Cytotoxic T-Cells attack the body cells that have been infected or are malignant and destroy them.
3. **Natural Killer (NK) Cells.** Unlike Cytoxic T-Cells, NK Cells do not need to recognize a specific invader to act. They attack a whole range of microbes in addition to tumor cells. Also, like Cytotoxic T-Cells, they kill enemy cells on contact by delivering lethal bursts of potent granular chemicals that "burn" holes in target cells causing them to leak and burst.

Phagocytes

Phagocytes are the large white cells that eat and digest (primarily through enzyme activity) invading pathogens. There are several kinds of phagocytes: monocytes, neutrophils, and macrophages. Macrophages, in particular, are especially fascinating and have a number of functions in the immune system. Not only do they attack foreign invaders; they also play a key role as scavengers by "eating up" worn out cells and other waste in the body.[3] And finally, once macrophages have "digested" an invader, they then present the key identifying molecules, or antigens, to the T-Cells to initiate the immune response.

Granulocytes

Granulocytes include eosiniphils, basophils, and neutrophils (neutrophils are classed as both phagocytes and granulocytes), and mast cells. Granulocytes destroy invaders by releasing granules filled with potent chemicals.

---

[1]T-Cells that cannot make this distinction are eliminated at this point so that they do not make their way into the body and begin attacking it.

[2]They are also called "suppressor cells."

[3]Macrophages play a key role in fasting. When you are not eating and creating new waste in the body, macrophages get a chance to get ahead of the game in terms of cleaning up the debris. Fasting time becomes spring cleaning time for macrophages.

Dendritic Cells

Dendritic cells are characterized by long threadlike tentacles that are used to wrap up not only antigens but expended lymphocytes and carry them to the lymph nodes for removal from the body.

The Organs of the Immune System

We've already discussed two key organs, the bone marrow (which produces the cells of the immune system) and the thymus (which trains the T-Cells). Other key organs include the lymph nodes, the spleen, the tonsils and adenoids, and the appendix. Although you can survive without some of these organs, they are vital and irreplaceable. Removal of any seriously compromises the immune system. The spleen, for example, serves as both a staging area for the white cell defenders and as a blood filtration plant for removing worn out blood cells. Removal of the spleen leaves one highly susceptible to infection. Even the tonsils and adenoids are not without unique value. There is some evidence to indicate that the only organs in the body that can produce a defense against polio are the tonsils and adenoids. If true, removal of these organs in children would make them more susceptible to polio.

The Complementary Immune System

At a certain point, when the macrophage immune system is totally overwhelmed, the "complementary immune system" kicks in. This secondary system is comprised of approximately 25 proteins/enzymes that activate in a cascading sequence and end with what's called the "membrane attack complex." As its name implies, this complex attacks the cell walls of invaders. A secondary function of the complementary immune system is to help rid the body of CIC's (circulating immune complexes) as discussed in Chapter 5. If the overload on the complementary immune system is great enough, severe inflammation of tissue, caused by the activity of albumins, can result. The bottom line is that the body's tissue literally begins to attack itself. That is to say, we now have an autoimmune condition!

How Your Immune System Communicates with Itself

We now have a sense of how the immune system works, how it identifies invaders and mounts a response, but how in the world does it communicate with itself? The answer lies in a set of powerful chemical messengers secreted by the cells of the immune system called cytokines. You've probably heard of several of these cytokines, including Interferon and Tumor Necrosis Factor; but it is the Interleukins which swarm through the body like billions of tiny messengers:

- Activating the B-Cells and T-Cells
- "Training" cells

- Promoting rapid growth of "trained" defenses
- Shutting down defenses when the threat is gone
- Controlling the inflammation response

In short, they provide a remarkable set of intelligent checks and balances on the immune system—guiding it, training it, regulating it, marshaling it as required, and resting it when no longer needed.

Building Immunity

Whenever T-Cells or B-Cells become activated by an invader, some of those cells become memory cells. That is, they encode a "memory" of the particular antigen associated with that invader so that the next time they encounter the same antigen, the immune system can respond without delay.

There are a number of factors that affect the level of immune response we are capable of mounting. Genetics certainly plays a role. Some individuals are just born with stronger immune systems than others. Diet, lifestyle, and environment can also enhance or erode the immune system. In addition, strength of immune response and the duration of immune memory are strongly influenced by the type of antigen involved, and how much of it originally entered the body.

When we are born, we have weak immune systems. Whatever immunity we have is given to us by our mothers. Almost immediately, however, assuming that we are nursing, that immunity begins to grow. The first "milk" we receive from mother is, in fact, not actually milk. It is a substance called colostrum, whose primary purpose is to jack up our immunity. Colostrum is packed with natural immune boosters such as lactoferrin, alkyglycerols, and transfer factor. In addition, as we discussed in Chapter 4, nursing helps build the probiotic cultures in the digestive tract, which also helps to build our immune systems.[1]

Vaccines

In the wisdom of modern medicine, we have created vaccines to "prebuild memory" for our immune systems—memory of significant diseases we have never had, such as measles, mumps, polio, diphtheria, small pox, etc. Vaccines contain a weakened sterilized version of microorganisms (or proteins from those microorganisms) that are capable of producing an immune response in the body without inducing a full-blown onset of the disease itself. Although vaccines have played a significant role in helping reduce the number of deaths among children, this benefit has not come without cost.

I'm not going to dwell on this issue, because I have a strong emotional attachment to it, which makes it impossible for me to be objective. My youngest

---

[1]Children that are put on formula are denied these benefits. Not only are formula fed children more liable to experience colic, ear infections and colds etc., but there is significant evidence that, for the most part, their immune systems never fully "catch up."

brother was one of those "small percentage" of children who responded badly to the series of three shots he received back in the early 60s. Each time he received one of the shots, he ran a high fever and cried all night—the last time literally screaming for several hours. Each time my mother called the pediatrician, who reassured her it was nothing to worry about. As it turns out, he was wrong. My brother, along with thousands of other children (Unfortunately, even a small percentage, when applied to a large number, still equals thousands of children), had an allergic reaction to the shots. Each shot caused a small brain hemorrhage, ultimately leaving him severely retarded. Although the manufacturer of the vaccine had indications that this was a possibility, they had not made it clear to the pediatricians who used it.[1] This sort of reaction to a vaccine and this sort of irresponsibility by a pharmaceutical company are not as anomalous as you might think.

- The polio vaccine that was given to children in the 50s and 60s was not as sterilized as originally thought. In fact, when better test equipment was later used, it was found that there were over **140 live viruses in those early versions of the polio vaccine.** With what result? Well for one thing, one of those viruses, SV 40, is strongly implicated in brain cancer.
- Jonas Salk testified before a Senate subcommittee that since 1961, except for a few importations from other countries, all cases of polio were caused by the Oral Polio Vaccine.[2]
- In 1986, the Federal Government set up a *National Vaccine Injury Compensation Program* to compensate vaccine-injured victims. **To date, close to $1 billion has been paid out.**
- In addition to the "active" part of the vaccine, the vaccine includes substances such as ethylene glycol (antifreeze), formaldehyde (a known carcinogen), and aluminum.

Look, I'm not saying vaccines should be eliminated—just that we should use a little more discrimination than we are at the moment. Eventually, it's possible that new techniques of genetic engineering, by being able to totally isolate the offending antigen, may be able to offer a safer form of vaccine. But until that day...

---

[1]Before 1990, doctors were not legally obligated to report adverse reactions to vaccines to the Center for Disease Control; and, even with the current legal obligation, it's estimated that only 10% of doctors report the damage they see to the CDC.

[2]In fact, there is strong evidence that the original polio epidemic itself in the late 1940s was caused by another vaccine. The early triple vaccine against diphtheria, whooping cough, and tetanus has been shown beyond doubt to cause paralytic polio in some children to whom it was administered. The incidence of polio in children vaccinated with this shot was statistically greater than in unvaccinated children. This scandal broke in Britain during 1949, an epidemic year for polio; other reports soon followed from Australia.

Problems That Can Occur with the Immune System

Problems that can occur are:

1. The Immune System is overwhelmed by too many invaders
2. The Immune System becomes weakened and vulnerable to attack
3. The Immune System becomes misprogrammed and loses the ability to identify invaders or mutated cells
4. The Immune System becomes misprogrammed and begins to mistakenly identify healthy body cells as the enemy and begins to attack them
5. The Immune System is compromised or missing some key component at birth

Of these problems, the first four are, in most cases, correctable. Only when the body is born without the ability to produce a key component are our options truly limited—but not necessarily hopeless.

Optimizing Your Immune System

Since the purpose of the body's immune system is to defend against attack and help initiate repair, the better it does it, the healthier we are. To facilitate this process, we need to address the two key areas of immune function we've already identified:

1. We have to improve overall immune function—to allow the body to better defend itself.
2. We need to specifically target (kill/destroy) invading bacteria, viruses, microorganisms and other related pathogens—to help out the immune system, as it were.

Scientists have known for years that it is possible to improve the functioning of the immune system. Here in the United States, the approach has been to use expensive, proprietary drugs. Current favorites include concentrated cytokines such as Interleukin and Interferon. The rest of the world, on the other hand, has adopted a more natural approach by seeking to use natural substances to:

- Stimulate and strengthen your immune system
- Fight infection
- Strengthen tissue against assault by invading microorganisms
- Stimulate macrophage capability
- Increase T-Cell production and protect T-helper cells

- Complement the action of Interferon and Interleukin 1
- Assist the Cell Mediated Immune Response

Surprisingly, not only are the natural immune boosters far safer than the drug approach (having far fewer side effects); they are also far more powerful than their pharmaceutical counterparts.

Let's take a look at some of the more powerful immune boosters available to us.

Echinacea

Echinacea is truly a miracle herb. For one thing, it contains echinacoside (a natural antibiotic, comparable to penicillin in effect) that can kill a broad range of viruses, bacteria, fungi, and protozoa, which makes it invaluable in wound healing and in the treatment of infectious diseases. Research has also reported echinacea's efficacy in treating colds, flu, bronchitis, tuberculosis, infections, etc.

Echinacea also contains echinacein, a biochemical that protects against germ attack by neutralizing the tissue dissolving enzyme, hyaluronidase, produced by many germs. Also, studies such as one published in *Infection and Immunology* show that echinacea contains substances that boost the ability of your body's macrophages to destroy germs. And other studies from the University of Munich have shown that echinacea extracts boost T-cell production by as much as 30% more than immune boosting drugs.

Pau d'arco

Pau d'arco (Tabebuia heptophylla) comes from the rain forests of Brazil and other areas of South America. This amazing herb nourishes the body's defense system and helps protect against pathogenic organisms. It has been used for centuries to improve immune function, detoxify, and reduce pain throughout the body—especially in the joints. Research has shown that it contains a natural antibacterial agent, has a healing effect on the entire body, cleanses the blood, and kills viruses.

Pau d'arco has been used as a treatment for AIDS, allergies, all infections and inflammations, anemia, asthma, arthritis, arteriosclerosis, as a blood builder, bronchitis, all types of cancer, candidiasis, colitis, cystitis, smoker's cough, diabetes, eczema, fistulas, gastritis, gonorrhea, hemorrhages, hernias, Hodgkin's disease, liver disease, leukemia, lupus, multiple sclerosis, osteomyelitis, Parkinson's disease, polyps, prostatitis, psoriasis, rheumatism, skin cancer, skin sores, spleen infections, snake bites, ulcers, varicose veins, warts, and plain old wounds.

Suma

Natives of the Amazon jungle have used Suma for at least the last 300 years. It wasn't until 1975, however, that Suma was introduced to the 20th century and tested at the University of Sao Paulo, Brazil.

The studies, conducted by Dr. Milton Brazzach, concluded that although it was not a cure, it nevertheless brought significant relief for cancer, diabetes, and gout sufferers—with no undesirable side effects. Since then, studies at the American College of the Healing Arts by Dr. Michael Tierra, author of *The Way of Herbs,* indicated that consistent use of Suma may help combat fatigue (including treatment of chronic fatigue and low-energy conditions), prevent colds and flus, speed healing, regulate blood sugar, and stimulate the sex drive.

The key working ingredients in Suma are:

- Pfaffic acid, which prevents the spread of various cell disorders.
- Pfaffocides and other saponins, which help stop diseases already in progress.
- The plant hormones sitosterol and stigmasterol, which prevent cholesterol absorption and improve blood circulation.
- Alantoin, which helps accelerate healing.
- And most important of all: Germanium. Suma has one of the highest concentrations of Ge-132 of any plant known.

What's the big deal with Ge-132? It was actually discovered about 20 years ago by a Japanese research chemist named Kazuhiko Asai. Its full name is bis-Carboxyethylgermanium Sesquioxide (or Germanium Sesquioxide, for short).

According to studies by Dr. Parris M. Kidd, "This substance, while free of major side effects, can apparently invigorate, rejuvenate, restore sexual function, protect against miscarriages during pregnancy, heal burns without scarring, cure radiation sickness, restore eyesight and hearing, kill the pain of advanced cancer, and shrink cancers within weeks. Circulatory disorders, including heart attacks, angina pectoris, stroke, and peripheral impairments respond well to Ge-132, as do hepatitis and cirrhosis and several behavior disorders."

Medicinal Mushrooms

Many of the compounds found in Reishi, Maitake, and Cordyceps mushrooms are classified as Host Defense Potentiators (HDP). It is believed that combinations of these compounds target and strengthen the human immune system as well as aid in neuron transmission, metabolism, hormonal balance and the transport of nutrients and oxygen. Through a host-mediated (T-cell) immune mechanism, they help the body regulate the development of lymphoid stem cells and other important defense responses.

- **Reishi:** The anti-cancer and immune enhancing effects of the Reishi mushroom are thought to be largely due to the polysaccharides. Reishi mushrooms are high in mucopolysaccharides, which your body incorporates into cellular membranes making them resistant to viruses and pathogenic bacteria. The polysaccharides appear to activate the macrophages, the white blood cell that "consumes" viruses, bacteria, and other large particulate matter.

- **Maitake** mushrooms have a very high concentration of a unique polysaccharide compound called beta 1,6 glucan, which researchers now consider to be one of the most powerful immune stimulants and adaptogens known. A research study reported in the *Chemical Pharmaceutical Bulletin* (1988) showed that maitake produced a 64% inhibition of breast cancer and tumor activity and a 75% inhibition of skin cancer and tumor activity. Also, laboratory studies conducted at the US. National Cancer Institute and the Japanese National Institute of Health showed that maitake extract kills the human immunodeficiency virus (HIV) and enhances the activity of T-helper cells. Research has demonstrated that Maitake simulates a variety of different immune cells including macrophages, NK-cells, Th, Tc and Tdh Cells. And not only does it stimulate the production of these immune cells, but it increases their efficiency and effectiveness by increasing the production of interleukin-l, interleukin-2, and lymphokines. As we've already talked about, these are chemicals that your body normally produces to stimulate the body's immune responses and help target foreign substances. Maitake has been confirmed to have a multifaceted benefit for cancer and tumors.
  - It protects healthy cells from becoming cancerous.
  - It helps prevent the spread of cancer (metastasis).
  - It slows or stops the growth of tumors.
  - It works in conjunction with chemotherapies by lessening their negative side effects. One study reported a 90% lessening of side effects from chemo including hair loss, pain and nausea.

- **Cordyceps** has properties similar to those of ginseng and has been used to strengthen and rebuild the body after exhaustion or long-term illness. It has also been used traditionally for impotence, neurasthenia, and backache. Recent research with extracts of Cordyceps has yielded a protein-bound polysaccharide with high oral activity against tumors, as well as immunological enhancement. Cordyceps is one of the most valued medicinal fungi in all Chinese medicine, and also one of the most expensive (costing as much as $249 per kilogram). Cordyceps is widely employed to treat upper respiratory problems, impotence, weakened immune systems, and by athletes to increase endurance.

Garlic

Garlic is one of the best infection fighters available for both bacterial and viral infections. One of its many ingredients, allicin,[1] is a natural antibiotic that does

[1]The same component that gives garlic its strong odor is the one that destroys, or inhibits various bacteria and fungi. The component is allicin, and when crushed, combines with the enzyme allinase and results in antibacterial action equivalent to 1% penicillin.

not appear to create resistant bacteria strains. In addition, fresh garlic extract has been shown to be deadly to many viruses.

Garlic also possesses the ability to stimulate the activity of the macrophages which engulf foreign organisms, such as viruses, bacteria, and yeast. Furthermore, garlic increases the activity of the T-helper cells. And garlic may be particularly effective in treating upper respiratory viral infections due to its immune-enhancing properties and its ability to clear mucous from the lungs. And finally, garlic is also effective against strep and staph bacteria.

(Everything that's been said about garlic goes for onions. Onions and garlic share many of the same powerful sulfur bearing compounds that work so effectively as antiviral and antibacterial agents.)

Aloe Vera

The polysaccharide component of aloe vera, acemannan, possesses significant immune enhancing and antiviral activity. Unfortunately, there is great variation in the amount of acemannan from one manufacturer to the next. Products with high levels of acemannan activity have been proven to increase lymphocyte response to alloantigen by enhancing the monocyte release of interleukin-I. In addition, acemannan has been shown to increase macrophage levels and have a positive effect on CD-4, CD-8, T-4, and T-8 levels.

Alkyglycerols

Alkyglycerols (also known as alkolxyglycerols, or AKG's) are naturally manufactured in the body and are found in mother's milk, the liver, the spleen, and bone marrow. They play a major role in the production and stimulation of white blood cells. They also help to normalize bone marrow function. The immune supportive effect of AKG's helps our bodies protect against bacterial, fungal, and viral infections.The most potent source of AKG's in the world is shark liver oil.

Lactoferrin

Lactoferrin is one of the cytokines produced in the human body. It is found anywhere that is especially vulnerable to attack, such as in the gut, eyes, ears, nose, throat, urinary tract, etc. Lactoferrin has been shown to:

- Inhibit virus replication, inlcuding both the AIDS and Herpes viruses, into healthy cells
- Inhibit tumor growth and metastasis
- It is directly toxic to both bacteria and yeast and is therefore invaluable in helping prevent bacterial and candida overgrowth in the gut
- Activate neutrophil cells

Supplementation with lactoferrin (or stimulating its production in your body with probiotics) can significantly boost the immune system and/or help the body recover from any existing infection. On the other hand, maintaining healthy levels of intestinal flora allow the body to produce its own lactoferrin.

Glutathione

Glutathione is a natural amino-acid-based tripeptide molecule found in human cells. In addition to being a powerful antioxidant,[1] glutathione works to support the active functioning of the immune system and is a key component of all lymphocytes. In fact, all lymphocytes require sufficient levels of intracellular glutathione to function properly. It also plays a major protective role against the damaging effects of the whole range of pathogens and carcinogens. For many people, glutathione supplements are upsetting to the stomach. Alternatives include the glutathione precursors cystine and glutamyl-cystine and specially formulated whey products.

Beta Glucan

Beta 1-3/1-6 Glucan is a natural complex carbohydrate found primarily in the cell walls of yeast. It works by "activating" macrophage cells.

General Recommendations

Too many people think of the immune system as something existing in isolation. That's a huge mistake. Let's take a quick walk through the Baseline of Health program and see how each system impacts the entire body.

- How good can your immune system be (taking all the supplements in the world that you want) if your colon is packed with 20 pounds of old fecal matter? A substantial portion of your immune system then has to combat the effects of self-toxicity. Clean up your intestinal tract, and you free up your immune system.
- Beneficial bacteria (if they're present) manufacture potent immune boosters such as Transfer Factor and Lactoferrin right in your intestinal tract. In other words, use a good probiotic and you substantially boost your immune system by increasing internal production of a number of powerful immune factors.
- As discussed in Chapter 5, supplementing with digestive enzymes significantly reduces the incidence of Circulating Immune Complexes, thus taking enormous stress off the complementary immune system.

---

[1] Glutathione is not unique in this regard. Many other natural substances, such as Vitamin C for example, also function as both antioxidants and immune boosters.

- Proper diet and nourishment boost your immune system. Each and every immune cell in your body is manufactured from the food you eat. A nutritionally deficient diet means functionally deficient immune cells. A good vitamin/mineral supplement enhances the production of your body's immune cells.
- The **Omega-9+** fatty acid is an immune system modulator that helps to keep the immune system properly programmed so it doesn't attack itself.
- A good full-spectrum antioxidant boosts the immune system in multiple ways. Just one example is Curcumin. In *Immunological Investigations*, 1999, Vol. 28, Issues 5–6, pp 291–303, there are published studies that prove that Curcumin can increase white blood cell count by some 50% in just 12 days—not to mention circulating antibodies by some 512 in the same time frame.
- Cleaning out the liver with an effective flush and rebuild program improves the liver's ability to produce immune factors and remove bacteria from the blood. Cleaning out the blood with an herbal blood cleanser and balancing your blood's pH also helps to improve immune function.
- And of course, **daily use of formulations comprised of the herbs discussed in this chapter has been proven to significantly enhance the immune system across the board**—even in the face of aggressive chemotherapy.
  - **Immune Boosters:** Echinacea, Pau d'arco, Suma, Reishi, Maitake, Cordyceps
  - **Pathogen Destroyers:** Garlic, Onion, Ginger, Habenero juice, Horseradish, Apple cider vinegar
- The mental exercises and visualizations outlined in the next chapter can double immune function in as little as 24 hours. In addition, the use of an herbal nerve tonic can dramatically reduce stress levels in the body, resulting in a dramatic increase in immune function—virtually overnight.
- And keep in mind that the primary entry point for most pathogens is via the eyes, nose, and mouth through contact with the hands. Keep in mind that the hands pick up potential threats by virtue of contact with other people (shaking hands, for example) and through contact with objects such as doorknobs and telephones. Regular washing of the hands throughout the day (even with regular soap) can serve to take a considerable amount of stress off of the immune system.
- And finally, one of the primarily benefits of regular exercise is an optimized immune system.

CHAPTER 15

THE THOUGHT THAT KILLS

For years stress and/or depression have been suspected of somehow increasing the risk of contracting numerous infectious diseases. In addition, there is mounting statistical evidence that increased levels of stress and depression also correlate with an increased incidence of cancer. And finally, there is strong statistical evidence linking stress and depression with death itself. Now, there is a new field of research, called pyschoneuroimmunology that is dedicated to unlocking the connection between our thoughts (i.e. our nervous systems) and our immune systems.

PSYCHONEUROIMMUNOLOGY

Researchers have discovered several links between our thoughts and our immune systems:

- For one, we know that when we are stressed, our bodies produce more adrenaline. And while it is true that adrenaline helps to mobilize the body's energy reserves, it's also true that adrenaline causes a decrease in available antibodies and a reduction in both the number and strength of lypmphocytes.
- We have also learned that the brain is directly wired to the organs of the immune system (the spleen, thymus, lymph nodes, and bone marrow) and that stress and depression affect their performance.
- But most interesting of all is the connection between the neuropeptides produced by brain cells and the rest of the body. In much the same way that the immune system uses the Interleukins to communicate with itself, the brain uses the hormone-like neuropeptides to communicate with itself **and** the rest of the body, including the immune system. The cells of the immune system carry receptors for the various neuropeptides produced by the brain. When we are happy, for example, the brain produces one kind of neuropeptide. The cells of the immune system have specific receptors for these "up" chemicals. Once received, these neuropeptides literally cause the immune system to strengthen and build. Correspondingly, when we are depressed, we produce a different set of neuropeptides. Immune cells also have receptors for these "down" communicators, whose net effect on the immune system is to shut it down.

Incidentally, this is by no means a one-way communication. The cells of the brain have receptor sites for the interleukins and interferon produced by the lymphocytes of the immune system. Even better, it turns out that some macrophages and activated lymphocytes actually are capable of producing their own neuropeptides—to communicate directly with the brain in its own language.

Beyond Psychoneuroimmunology

Basically, through the same two systems (the nervous system and the circulatory system) that our mind interacts with our immune system, our mind also connects with every organ and cell in our body, affecting the performance, functioning, growth, etc. of our:

- Immune system
- Bones
- Bone marrow
- Glands
- Heart (everything from heart rate to the heart tissue itself)
- The walls of our veins and arteries
- The functioning of individual cells in the body
- Even, as we will see, the very structure of our DNA

The entire body is literally created and run by the brain—with equal input back from the organs and cells themselves, again through both the direct wired connections of the nervous system and the neuropeptides traveling through the circulatory system. The net result is that in addition to what medical researchers have been able to verify and explain, there are a number of "incidents" that hint at so much more.

Depression and Heart Attacks

A group of medical researchers in Montreal tracked 222 post heart attack victims, both men and women. The researchers found that those who were depressed (who felt sad, hopeless, and listless) were more likely to die of another heart attack within 18 months of their first heart attack than those who were not—**10 times more likely, in fact.**

The January '95 issue of the *American Journal of Medicine* reported on a study of patients with a history of heart disease that found that those who were depressed were eight times more likely to develop potentially deadly heart rhythms than those who were not depressed.

A 10-year study was conducted to follow the mortality rates of people who had experienced stroke. Those who had been diagnosed with either major or minor depression were 3.4 times as likely to have died within the follow-up period. The death rate among depressed patients with few social contacts was especially high—over 90%!

In a study of 194 heart attack patients, those who reported lower amounts of emotional support were nearly 3 times more likely to die within 6 months than those with higher levels of emotional support.

The Monday Morning Blahs

Have you ever wondered when most people die? Statistically, it turns out that people are more likely to die on Monday morning before going to work than at any other time of the week. There has been much speculation as to why this happens; but in general, most people agree it's something along the lines of: "Most people have heart attacks on Monday morning, because they are stressed that they are heading back to jobs they can't stand after a weekend off."

Placebos

On average, 35% of all people who receive a given placebo experience a significant effect.

Idle Chatter in the Operating Room

For years it has been suspected by many doctors (and pooh poohed by many more) that patients under anesthesia can hear their surgeon's comments, and that what they hear affects them. There were many anecdotal stories of doctors, who upon opening a patient up, would see a tumor and comment out loud that it looked malignant. And then, even though the tumor would later prove to be nonmalignant, the patient nevertheless would fade rapidly and be dead in a matter of days.

Well, new studies are now proving that not only is this true, but to a degree far higher than previously imagined. Dr. Henry Bennett, a psychologist from the University of California Medical School at Davis, suggests that, under anesthesia, patients might be **especially** vulnerable to upsetting remarks they overhear since their normal coping techniques aren't available to them. Specifically, the studies that support this statement include:

- A number of patients were given the suggestion during surgery that one of their hands was becoming warmer and the other cooler. The temperature of both hands changed accordingly.
- In another study, patients were played a taped message while they were anesthetized during surgery that told them that if they heard the same message later, they should signify that they heard it by touching their ears in a postoperative interview. Later, in the interview, all of the patients absentmindedly tugged

at their ears—although not one of the patients could recall having heard the message.

- During back surgery, which normally causes urination problems for the patients after surgery, researchers suggested to the anesthetized patients that they would be able to relax their pelvic muscles after the surgery, and thus would need no catheter. None of the patients who received the suggestion subsequently needed a catheter.

DNA

In 1952, the *British Medical Journal* reported on an extraordinary case[1] concerning Brocq's disease, a genetic disorder that causes the skin to resemble the scales of a reptile.[2] What was so extraordinary about this case is that although Brocq's disease is an hereditary genetic condition, and considered incurable by the medical community, it was nevertheless cured in this particular case through hypnosis. To put it simply, under hypnosis, the patient, a 16-year-old boy, was able to "go in" and literally reprogram his DNA. The net result is that within 10 days of starting treatment, the boy was symptom free—and remained so for at least 5 years, at which point his therapist lost touch with him.

Cancer

A now well-known example was reported by Dr. Bruno Klopfer in the *Journal of Projective Techniques* back in 1957. A patient of Dr. Klopfer's, whose cancer had metastasized and whose body was riddled with tumors, had reached the point where all available medical approaches had failed, and he was confined to bed with only a few days to live. Then, just before the end, the patient heard about Krebiozen, an experimental drug then being tested. Desperate, he demanded that his doctors include him in the experimental trials. Believing that the man was as good as dead anyway, and that they therefore had nothing to lose, they put him on Krebiozen. Miraculously, the man's tumors began to melt away. He made a remarkable recovery and was discharged from the hospital.

Two months later, however, reports began to appear that continuing research on Krebiozen had raised serious doubts about the efficacy of the drug. Within a few days of the patient's reading these reports, his tumors had returned and he was once again on the verge of terminal. At this point, his doctor did something unusual in the medical profession—he lied to his patient. He told the man that they now had available a newer and more potent version of Krebiozen. He then proceeded to inject the man, not with a new and improved version of Krebiozen, not even with the original version, but with plain old water. Astoundingly, the

---

[1]A.A. Mason, "A Case of Congenital Ichthyosiform," *British Medical Journal.* (1952), pp. 422-423.

[2]Many so-called "alligator people" in circus sideshows are victims of Brocq's disease.

man's tumors once again began to melt away. As before, the man made a remarkable recovery and went home.

He then remained perfectly healthy, in full remission for seven whole months, until he saw a news report that declared "Nationwide AMA Tests Show Krebiozen to Be Worthless as a Cancer Treatment." Two days later, he was dead!

Stress and Depression

For years, stress and/or depression have been suspected of increasing the risk of contracting numerous infectious diseases. In addition, there is mounting statistical evidence that increased levels of stress and depression also correlate with an increased incidence of cancer. And finally, there is strong statistical evidence linking stress and depression with death itself.

Stress

Stress is your body's response to all of the demands made upon it. Your body responds to all stresses, both positive and negative, by trying to get back to normal.

- 43% of all adults suffer adverse health effects due to stress.
- 75-90% of all visits to primary care physicians are for stress-related complaints or disorders.

When a stressor is perceived, the hypothalamus triggers your adrenal glands to release corticosteroids to increase metabolism to provide an immediate increase in energy. Simultaneously, your pituitary releases a hormone called ACTH, which causes your adrenal glands to release epinephrine and norepinephrine, which work to prolong your body's fight-or-flight response.

If a stressful situation goes on for too long without any relief, you may feel tired, irritable, depressed, or anxious. You may have trouble sleeping or eating, or you might experience diseases and disorders, such as headaches, insomnia, high blood pressure, and cardiovascular and kidney diseases, colds, ulcers, asthma, heart attack, and/or stroke.

- Stress has been linked to all the leading causes of death, including heart disease, cancer, lung ailments, accidents, cirrhosis, and suicide.
- Stress is said to be responsible for more than half of the 550 million workdays lost annually because of absenteeism.

Eventually, your body's energy reserves are exhausted; it breaks down. Recent research has confirmed the role of stress in cardiovascular disease, cancer, gastrointestinal, skin, neurologic and emotional disorders, and a host of disorders linked to immune system disturbances, ranging from the common cold and herpes, to arthritis, cancer, and AIDS.

Depression

Depression works on your body in different ways than stress, but the results are the same.

Your body is a product of your thoughts. The cells of your body have receptor sites for the various neuro-hormones you produce. Your immune cells, to use just one example, have receptor sites for each of those hormones. When you are happy, you produce a set of neuro-hormones that are picked up by the cells of your immune system. These particular neuro-hormones tell your immune system to jack up—which it does. In other words, happy thoughts improve your health. However, when you are depressed, the opposite happens. The neuro-hormones your body produces literally shut down your immune system. In effect, negative thoughts can actually kill you.

The Pharmaceutical Solution - SSRIs

The major pharmaceutical companies, as usual, have developed a set of drugs called selective serotonin reuptake inhibitors (SSRIs) to "manage the symptoms" associated with stress and depression. You might know them as Prozac®, Zoloft®, Paxil®, Luvox®, Celexa®, Effexor® and Serzone®.

Thanks to millions and millions of dollars in promotion, some misguided books that jumped on the bandwagon, and our own marvelous tendency to believe in magic bullets, we have become a "Prozac Nation." But not without cost.

- SSRIs cause mania and delusions of grandeur in one out of every 25 children taking the drugs.
- A tendency to violence has been reported in 1 out of 16 SSRI users
- In 70% of all murder/suicides involving women and children, the women were on SSRIs

The Colombine Tragedy, et al

- Specialized testing during the autopsy of Eric Harris, one of the Colombine shooters, showed "therapeutic" levels of an SSRI in his blood. In addition, he was also taking cough syrup. The interaction between cough medications containing dextromethorphan (found in Robitussin, for example) and the SSRIs can greatly increase the possibility of a toxic reaction known as serotonin syndrome leading to PCP (Angel Dust) reactions. In effect, Eric Harris was unknowingly on the equivalent of Angel Dust. That explains a lot.
- Kip Kinkle, who shot his parents and then shot his classmates in Oregon, was on SSRIs.
- Brynn Hartmann, the actor Phil Hartmann's wife, was on SSRIs when she shot her husband and committed suicide.

- In March of 1998, Matthew Beck went on a bloody rampage at his office, the Connecticut Lottery Corp. headquarters, killing four senior lottery officials before committing suicide. He was on 2 antidepressants, including Luvox.
- Many children under the age of 3 have already been given Prozac.
- Special "flavored" SSRIs are now in development just for children.

The Herbal Solution

For the vast majority of people bothered by stress or depression, there is a safe, effective solution.

A well-designed herbal formula made from high-quality herbs and that makes use of the complementary synergies inherent in many herbs can prove remarkably effective. Look for an herbal formula that contains herbs such as:

- **Valerian root.** For centuries, Valerian has been used to treat nervous tension and panic attacks. A wonderful herb, Valerian is calming and quieting to the nervous system.
- **Kava kava** is the herb of choice to relax the body, relieve stress, to combat mild to moderate anxiety, for relief from headache and back pain. Kava is now recognized by many doctors as an alternative to drugs like Xanax and Valium.
- **Lobelia** is an extremely powerful anti-spasmodic and sedative. It helps improve breathing dramatically by dilating the bronchial tubes—great for asthmatics.
- **Passionflower** is remarkably effective as a sedative to calm nerves that get on edge.
- **St. John's wort.** Sometimes called "Nature's Prozac," St. John's wort helps relieve stress, anxiety, and tension. In Germany, it is the most popular antidepressant, outselling Prozac 3-1.
- **Black cohosh.** First used by the American Indians, Black cohosh works to soothe the body by reducing the rapidity of the pulse. Black cohosh also works internally to help soothe any nervous disease or spasm.
- **Skullcap, Hops, and Catnip.** Three herbs that have a long history as marvelously effective herbal tranquilizers, sedatives, and sleep aids.

Other Solutions

For the vast majority of people, the above type of herbal formulation will prove all that is needed to help relax, pick up one's spirits, and sleep the sleep of angels.

For an added boost, some people might wish to add one or both of the following.

- **5-HTP**

  5-hydroxytryptophan, a more active form of l-tryptophan, can provide a low-cost boost to the herbal formula described above.

- **SAMe**

  200–400 mg of SAMe (S-adenosyl-methionine, which is made from substances naturally found in your body) twice a day on an empty stomach can be extremely helpful in alleviating depression. Unfortunately, SAMe is very expensive, costing anywhere from $2 to $15 a day.

General Recommendations

Casting aside the extreme point of view that all illness originates in the mind ("Harriett, why are you choosing to give yourself breast cancer?"), we are nonetheless left with the fact that what we think (and how we think) does absolutely (and unequivocally) affect our health. Or as Dr. John Christopher, one of America's foremost naturopaths, was fond of saying, **"Most people need a colonic between the ears."**

The bottom line is that if you want to make your mind your partner in health, you need to work at it. **It takes work to move your mind out of stress and/or depression.** Listed below are four exercises to help you begin the process.

- **Learn to Meditate.** If nothing else, just try watching your breath. Sit down. Keep your back straight. Close your eyes and watch your breath. Watch as your breath goes in and your lungs fill. Watch as it goes out and your lungs empty. Don't force; just watch.

- **Learn to Visualize.** After you've meditated for a few minutes and calmed down, practice a visualization. See your body as made of healing light. Imagine the light penetrating and healing every cell in your body. If you are sick, focus the light on the diseased area.

- **Practice Affirmation.** What we say matters. We all know, for example, someone who uses the word "afraid" all the time. As in:
  - "I'm afraid I won't be able to go tonight."
  - "I'm afraid I've eaten too much; I'm absolutely stuffed."
  - "I'm afraid I'm almost out of gas."
  - etc.

- Is it any wonder that eventually they're afraid all the time? And then there are the examples that Dr. Bernie Siegal includes in his book *Love, Medicine, and Miracles,* such as:

- •• The man who said "he was always considered spineless" and in the end developed multiple myeloma in his backbone to support his contention.
- •• Or the woman who had had a mastectomy who told Dr. Siegel that she "needed to get something off her chest."

- The bottom line is that instead of being controlled by the things we say, instead of having our health compromised by idle words, we should put words to work for us. Try repeating to yourself over and over with each step you take when you walk, or while you're driving something like:
  - •• "I'm joy. I'm peace. I'm health. I'm light." Or make up your own. If so, make it short and rhythmical, so it sort of says itself to a walking cadence. It really does work magic. I once hiked the full length of the John Muir Trail, about 237 miles, silently reciting a similar affirmation every single step of the way. By the end of the trip, I had repeated the affirmation something over 500,000 times—and I was sailing up and down over 10,000 foot passes and up and down the 15,000 feet of Mt. Whitney.

- Take an herbal break. Use an herbal nerve-tonic formulation that contains herbs such as Valerian Root, Kava kava,[1] Passionflower, Hops, Black cohosh, St. John's wort, and Lobelia.

---

[1]There have been several reports in the press recently claiming that Kava kava may cause liver damage. These reports are based on tainted evidence from Europe and totally erroneous data from the FDA Medwatch site. The bottom line is that the issues of kava's safety and efficacy have been studied extensively, including a statistical review of seven human clinical trials, published in the *Journal of Clinical Psychopharmacology*, which indicated no significant adverse effects related to kava use and liver toxicity.

Chapter 16

Exercise: Move or Die

No one likes to hear this, but it's true. If you don't move, you die. Exercise fundamentally changes every system and function in your body.

Circulation

First and foremost, exercise is about circulation—and not just blood circulation, but every circulation system in the body.

Blood

Exercise definitely improves the flow of blood. Think what this means for a moment. Even if you eat healthy foods and partake of the most powerful supplements in the world, if that nutrition can't easily reach some part[1] of your body because circulation is restricted, then that part will suffer, waste away, and become diseased. If the blockage is total, that part will die.

Blood also brings oxygen to and removes carbon dioxide waste from every cell and organ in your body. Again, if circulation is restricted, the cell or organ slowly suffocates in its own waste. And finally, blood carries immune cells and pH balancers into every part of your body. Exercise literally drives your blood through your body, forcing oxygen and nutrition into every nook and cranny.

Lymph

Back in Chapter 3, we talked about how your lymph is your body's sewer system, removing dead cells, waste, toxic matter, heavy metals, bacteria, etc. from body tissue. Unfortunately, the lymph system has no pump of its own. To a large degree, your body depends on muscle movement to press waste through the lymph system. If you don't move, your lymph is stagnant; you end up poisoning yourself; you die. (Keep in mind that this statement is both absolute and relative. In other words, it's definite that stagnant lymph will ultimately destroy your health, but the process may take a number of years in some people.)

---

[1]This could be an organ, a group of cells within an organ, or even one single cell.

Heart

The heart is a muscle and grows stronger with exercise.

Blood Pressure

Exercise lowers blood pressure.

Colon

Exercise is a key factor in promoting peristalsis and relieving constipation.

Bones

Exercise increases bone density.

Cancer

As the *New England Journal of Medicine* reported in their May 1, 1997 issue, women who exercise regularly reduce their risk of breast cancer by 72%.

Strength

Strength is not just for showing off in the weight room. It is essential as we get older. People who exercise regularly are far less likely to fall and break bones. Not only because the exercise has made them stronger, but also because the exercise gave them better balance and because the larger muscle mass cushions the bones better and protects them.

Body Fat

There's nothing more fundamental to losing body fat than exercise. Not, as many people think, because the exercise burns the fat off, but rather, because muscle burns fat even while you sleep. The more muscle you have, the more calories you burn. Sixty to 70% of the energy your muscles burn (even while sleeping) is fat. Every pound of muscle that you have burns fat calories 24 hours a day. Think about that. If you add 4 pounds of muscle to your body, every day you automatically burn an extra 200 calories or so, free of charge (plus another 200 calories from your exercise).

Energy

The Chinese call it Chi; the yogis of India call it Prana; here in the States, people call it Life Force. Whatever you call it, it can be seen, measured, photographed, felt, and manipulated. According to Chinese medicine, restriction in its flow is the ultimate cause of all disease. Exercise stimulates and helps move this "energy" through blocked areas of the body.

Biochemical Changes

Exercise produces "happy" biochemicals called endorphins. Sometimes called "the runner's high," these endorphins drive away stress and depression and stimulate the immune system.

In addition, exercise increases levels of human growth hormone (the youth hormone) in the body. Aerobic exercise can increase HGH levels by as much as 200%. Weight training can increase HGH levels an astounding 400%.

Strength Benefits

Everyone thinks of strength training as a young person's activity, but in fact, the older you are, the more benefits it provides.

- As reported in the *Journal of the American Medical Association,* two 45-minute weight (strength) training sessions a week can improve bone density, muscle mass, strength, balance, and physical activity in older women (ages 50–70). **After one year of strength training, women emerged physiologically younger by 15–20 years than when they began.** Other studies have demonstrated the same results for men who weight train.
- **People in their 70s and 80s can experience strength gains of as much as 180% in a matter of just a few weeks.**

General Recommendations

Actually, you need to cross-train for maximum benefit. **You need to do aerobic exercise, weight training, and stretching.**

- **Aerobic** exercise should be practiced every other day. By definition, aerobic exercise:
  - Is continuous—nonstop.
  - Lasts at least 12 minutes—preferably 20 minutes or more. The key is to exercise longer, not harder.

- - Has a comfortable pace—not so fast that you can't talk during it if you want.
  - Involves your leg muscles.
- **Weight Training** should also be practiced every other day. Alternate your days with aerobic exercise. You can go to a gym or use a machine at home.
- **Stretching** should be done every day. It's invaluable as part of your aerobic and weight training sessions to prevent injuries. It's also great exercise on its own. In addition to helping prevent injuries, stretching also:
  - Lubricates your joints.
  - Squeezes lymph through your body.
  - Revitalizes the discs in your spine. Backbends, in particular, squeeze the discs like a sponge, so that when you release the stretch, the discs soak up water and fill up to their original size.
  - Rebounding is great exercise, particularly for moving lymph.
  - Yoga is spectacular exercise in that it stretches every part of your body and is renowned for its ability to relieve stress and depression. I can't recommend it highly enough.

CHAPTER 17

IT'S ALL ABOUT ENERGY

All life is energy. Every nerve impulse in your body is an electric current. Our muscles are powered by chemical energy. Every cell in your body is a mini-battery pumping out 70–90 millivolts when healthy.

The steak and potatoes that you eat for dinner are really just fuel for the fire. Eating is like throwing coal in a furnace. Digestion is nothing more than a slow form of burning that produces energy for your body to live on. In fact, death itself is defined as the absence of electrical activity in the brain. In the end, all life is energy.

Optimize that Energy and You Optimize Your Health.

Energy is neither good nor bad; it just is. The same electricity that is used by a chiropractor or a physical therapist to stimulate your muscles and promote healing with a TENS machine is the same electricity that is used in prisons to execute people in electric chairs. So, is electricity good or bad? The answer is neither. It's just a question of what frequency and amplitude you use and how you use it.

Charge Your Body with the Right Frequencies and You Prevent Disease.

The same laser light that is used to shoot down enemy missiles or as a death ray in a movie is also used by your eye-doctor to improve your vision via Lasik surgery or by your plastic surgeon to remove facial hair and wrinkles. Again, the difference is merely one of frequency and amplitude.

The proper use of energy in the healing arts has a long and significant history. From the TENS machines and laser surgery that we've already mentioned to the use of sound waves to break up kidney stones, or X-rays and magnetic fields to see into the body and the use of light to clean the blood.

Some forms of energy are more effective than others.

As we will see, scalar energy is merely another application of healing energy. It is the application of science as nature intended.

A New Paradigm

We are about to talk about some things concerning health and nutrition that are probably brand new to you. This topic is not inherently difficult to understand, but since it represents a total paradigm shift in how you will look at health and nutrition, we will have to proceed slowly.

We're going to learn how to actually embed healing energy in nutritional products.

Also, in order to explain everything, we will have to touch on some very esoteric areas such as higher mathematics and subatomic particles. Don't panic. It won't be too involved, and after every difficult section, I will summarize what you just read and tell you the key points you need to remember.

We're also going to learn how healing energy frequencies are transferred from the products you ingest into every single cell of your body, with profound implications for your overall health.

With that said, let's begin.

The Nature of Energy

All of the energy that we normally think of is characterized by both particle and wavelike properties. The waveform of all these energies can be graphed as a hertzian wave (either in the form of a sine wave or a step wave).

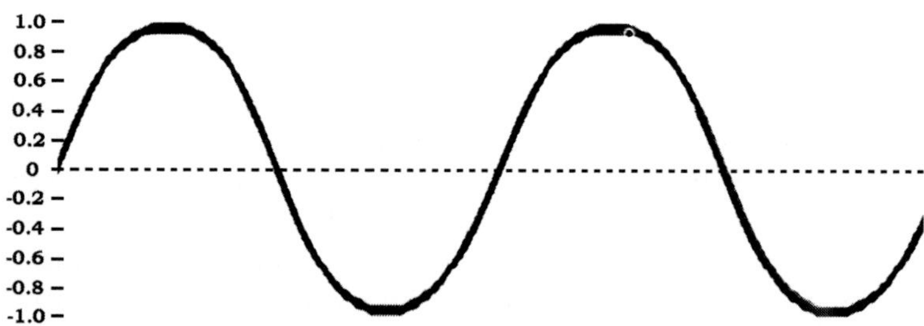

We're talking about everything from electricity to magnetism, from light to sound. The only difference between all of these forms of energy is how fast the waves rise and fall (the frequency) and how intense those rises and falls are (their amplitude).

SCALAR ENERGY

Several years ago, I discovered and developed the Barron Effect, which incorporates the principle of energy enhancement to modify the physical structure of herbs during the tincture manufacturing process. The net result is herbal tinctures that are over 100% stronger than anything the world has previously seen. In a sense, the use of scalar energy to enhance the effectiveness of nutritional products is an extension of that effect—but at the same time is an entirely different animal. Understand, scalar energy has existed since the beginning of time; however, it's only recently that scientists have discovered and begun to make use of it.

It was actually back in the mid 1800s that the existence of scalar energy was first proposed in a series of 4 groundbreaking equations by the Scottish mathematician, James Clerk Maxwell.

$$\nabla \times H = \varepsilon_0 \, \delta E/\delta t + j$$

$$\nabla \times E = - \mu_0 \, \delta H/\delta t$$

$$\nabla \cdot H = 0$$

$$\nabla \cdot E = \rho/\varepsilon_0$$

Don't even think about trying to understand these equations.

- Just as a minor reference, H refers to the magnetic field. E refers to the energy field. Most of the other symbols are Greek letters such as epsilon and delta. The upside down triangle represents the Vector Differential.

But forget all of that. The key to these equations—what makes them remarkable in history is the use of the ***P*** symbol, which stands for Scalar Charge Density, thus representing the first time that the existence of scalar energy was theoretically proposed.

It was almost a half century later before Nicola Tesla was actually able to demonstrate the existence of scalar energy. When Tesla died, he took the secret of scalar generation with him, and it took almost another full century before science was once again able to demonstrate, positively, the existence of scalar energy and begin an exploration of its potential.

What are Scalar Waves?

The standard definition of scalar waves is that they are created by a pair of identical (or replicant) waves (usually called the wave and its antiwave) that are in phase spatially, but out of phase temporally. That is to say, the two waves are physically identical, but out of phase in terms of time. The net result is that scalar waves are a whole different animal from normal hertzian waves. They even look different—like an infinitely projected mobius pattern on axis.

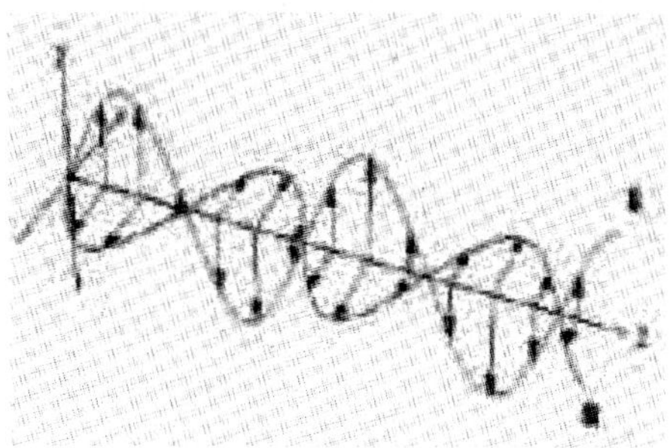

Different How?

Scalar energy is different from standard hertzian electromagnetic fields in a number of important ways.

- First, it's more field-like than wavelike. Instead of running along wires or shooting out in beams, it tends to "fill" its environment. **This becomes very important in terms of developing the technology for embedding products with scalar energy.**

- For many of the same reasons, it is capable of passing through solid objects with no loss of intensity. In fact, that is exactly what Tesla demonstrated over 100 years ago when he projected a scalar wave through the earth with no loss of field strength. **Again, this is vital in the development of technology capable of embedding scalar energy in products.**

- It implants its signature on solid objects. This is actually the heart of the issue. All electric fields can implant their signature on objects, but not to the degree that scalar energy can. **This becomes extremely important when we actually talk about the mechanics of embedding the energy field in products, and then transferring that charge from the products into every cell of your body.**

- Scalar energy can regenerate and repair itself indefinitely. This also has important implications for the body. In other words, **once the charge is implanted, you can keep it there with the regular ingestion of charged products.**

- **In fact, the right scalar frequencies have a whole range of profound beneficial effects on the human body. (And we will detail each and every one very shortly.)**

  In the "New Age" community there has been much talk of the benefit of things like Tachyons, Radionics, and Pyramids, etc. **Analysis shows that these are all, at heart, scalar generating devices—but cannot come close to the effectiveness of ingesting Scalar Enhanced™ products.**

Generating Scalar Energy

Actually, scalar waves can be generated in many ways. For example, you can generate them electronically, magnetically, physically, or optically (by the movement of phased patterns on a computer monitor). You can actually buy wristwatches that incorporate computer chips that generate protective scalar fields. The most interesting technology for generating scalar waves, however, has been developed by a group that includes several ex-NASA engineers.

Through the use of proprietary computer programs, they are able to cause both the computer's CPU to oscillate at predetermined frequencies and emit scalar energy, while at the same time generating scalar charges off of the computer monitor by running very precise hieroglyphic patterns on the monitor. To create what they call a charging chamber. They aim four monitors (precisely aligned with lasers) at an amplifying devise in the center of the room. The entire room then becomes a scalar charging chamber. This produces an intensity of charge and an ability to regulate frequency beyond any other comparable technology in use today. Any individual standing in the room is charged, and, as it turns out, so is any product or object—up to its ability to hold the charge. The higher the quality of the product (whole foods vs isolates, organic vs inorganic, etc.) the better that product is able to hold the charge.

Embedding Scalar Energy in Products

As I mentioned earlier, all life is fundamentally energy based, and therefore, all life has numbers of structures capable of holding a scalar charge. In point of fact, the very same structures that allow the scalar charge to be embedded in products also allow that charge to be transferred to the human body from those same products. For example:

- There are many crystalline structures in every cell wall—all capable of holding a charge
- There are many liquid crystal structures in the collagen network comprising all of the space between cells—also capable of holding a charge

And in Your Very DNA

We are going to get very abstract, for one final moment, before we begin to simplify everything and bring it all together. So just hang in there for a little longer.

There are Quantum Mechanical models that describe subatomic particles such as Excitons, Plasmons, and Solitons that can store and carry biological information along macromolecules in response to low-level scalar energy.

In other words, scalar energy is capable of imprinting itself on your very DNA.

Before we move on to the benefits of scalar energy for your health, it would be worth dwelling for a moment on what proof exists that everything I'm talking about is real.

There Is Proof

It is possible to measure scalar fields, but most people don't have the required equipment. Therefore, let's turn to a form of proof that we can see right now—Kirlian photography. A Kirlian photograph is merely a specialized kind of photography that images the bioelectric field that surrounds all objects—particularly living objects.

U.S. News and World Report ran an article some time ago calling Kirlian photography a hoax. To quote from the article:

> *"Controlled experiments have shown that the Kirlian photos (captured by passing an electric current through the subject, whose "energies" are then recorded on special photographic plates) are the result of moisture and pressure, not spiritual vitality."*

And that's absolutely true, **as far as it goes.** The simple fact is, though, that it's possible to set up a hermetically sealed environment where moisture and pressure are constant, and therefore not influencing the outcome of the pictures. And yet, even in those controlled environments, it's possible to produce startling and revealing photos. For example:

Here are two pictures of lentil sprouts, identical, except for the fact that the lentil on the left has been soaked in very hot water for a minute or so. According to the *U.S. News and World Report* article, since it has more moisture in it, it should conduct more electricity than the unblanched lentil on the right and produce a brighter field.

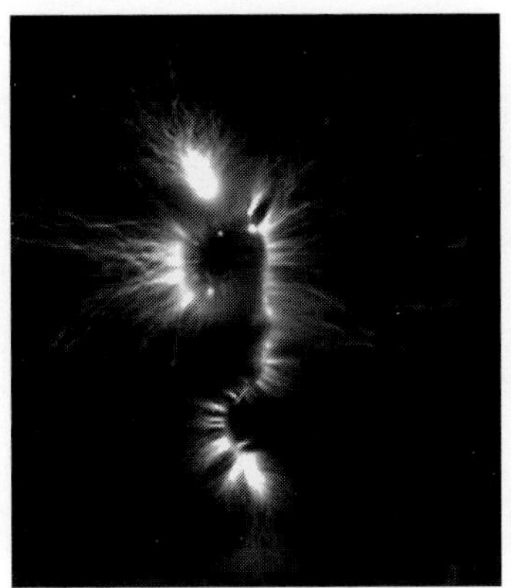

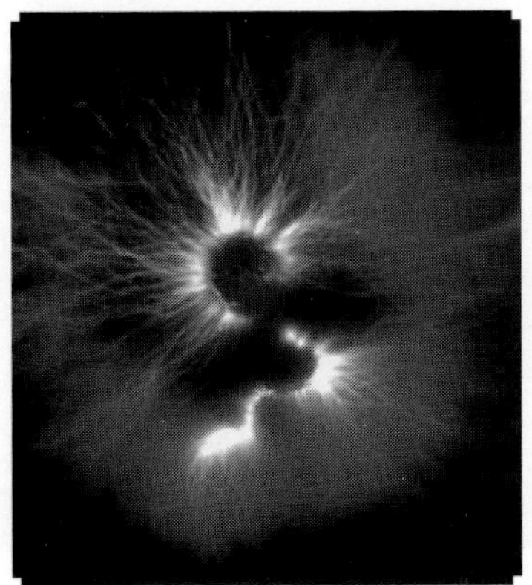

As you can see, the exact opposite is true. (If you're looking at a black and white printout, the greatly expanded red area appears dark gray.) And that's why the National Institute of Health and Cambridge University, among other major institutes, are studying Kirlian photography.

So what can we learn about Scalar Enhanced™ products through Kirlian photos? Well, the absolute most important thing we can learn is that the scalar charge is, unquestionably, embedding itself in the products. What follows are just a couple of examples of products before and after embedding.

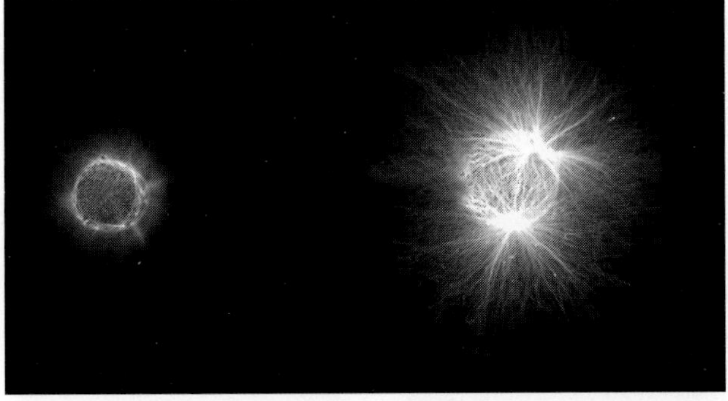

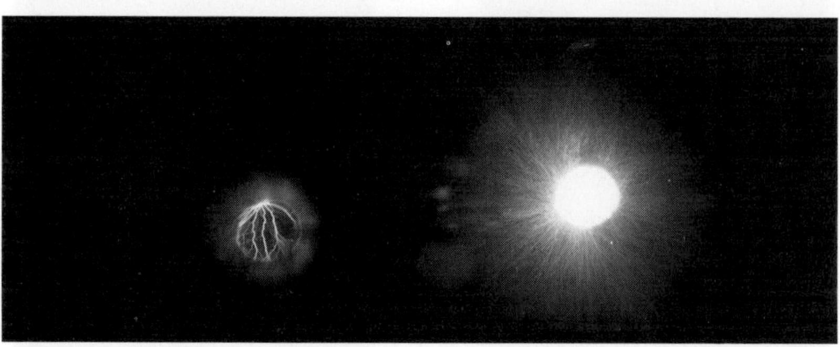

The two sets of photographs above, by themselves, are revolutionary in their implications. (Incidentally, these images were produced using a brand new process—side-by-side direct digital imaging, which even further diminishes the effect of outside factors such as moisture, temperature, and pressure.)

The bottom line is that experience tells us that the more alive something is (the more organic it is) the bigger its energy field will be. And Scalar Enhanced™ products always demonstrate a bigger field.

Benefits

This is the big question, isn't it? What health benefits are there to consuming Scalar Enhanced ™ products? As it turns out, they are many.

First of all, enhanced products are more assimilable by the body. They are absorbed better and faster. We actually can prove that enhanced products can be assimilated by your body and totally transform your bioelectric field in as little as 10 seconds. There are no other products in the world that can do that. Here is a set of pictures that image the body's bioelelectric field as registered through

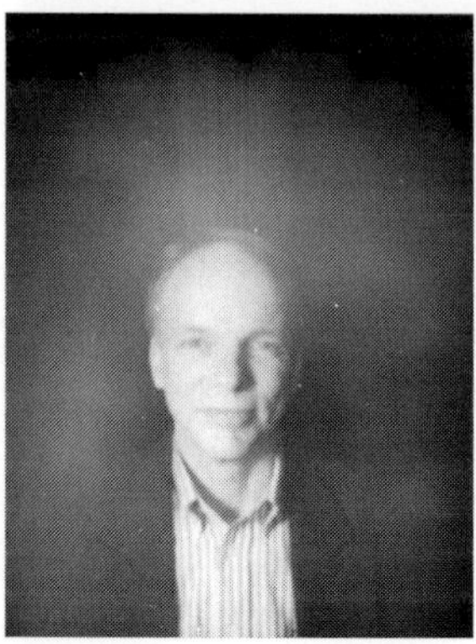

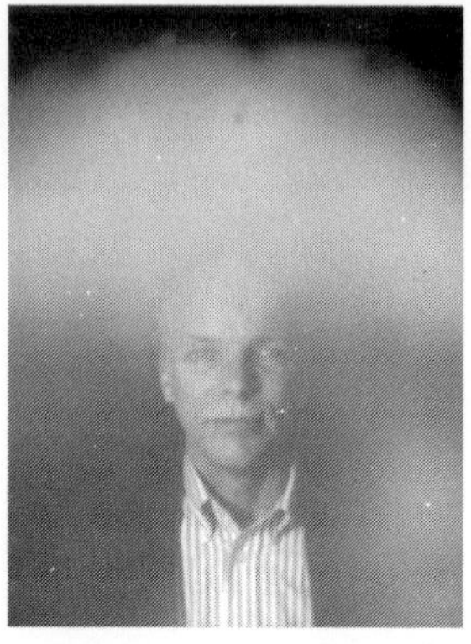

biofeedback devices that measure galvanic skin response and body temperature. What you are seeing is the field before taking any Scalar Enhanced™ product, and then the change in the field literally just 10 seconds after putting the enhanced product in your mouth.

Results this profound and this quickly realized have never before been seen—ever—by any nutritional products of any kind in the entire history of nutritional supplements. These pictures literally represent an entirely new standard in health and nutrition—a standard that every company will one day have to match.

But above and beyond that, the scalar charges that we embed in our products carry a whole range of benefits inherent in the charge itself—independent of the product. In that sense, the product functions as a carrier of the healing charge. There are at least a dozen major health benefits that come from this charge—**and they are profound.** Regular intake of Scalar Enhanced™ products can:

- Eliminate and nullify the effects of manmade frequencies (60 cps) in the human body.
- Increase the energy level of every single cell in the body to the ideal 70–90 millivolt range.
- Increase the energy covalent level of every single hydrogen atom in the body as verified by spectrographs. This is significant because covalent hydrogen bonds are what hold your DNA together. In other words, consuming Scalar Enhanced™ products can protect your DNA from damage.
- Improve cell wall permeability thus facilitating the intake of nutrients into each and every cell and the elimination of waste from each and every cell. (As a result of the high transmembrane potential mentioned above, Scalar Enhanced™ products effectively cause every single cell in your body to detox).
- Decrease the surface tension of the embedded products, thereby significantly reducing the time required for your body to assimilate those same products.
- Increase overall body energy levels as a result of increasing cellular energy for trillions of cells.
- Cleanse the blood improving chylomicron levels (protein/fat particles floating in the blood) and triglyceride profiles and fibrin patterns.
- Improve immune function by as much as 149% as proven in laboratory studies.
- Improve mental focus as demonstrated by increased amplitude of EEG frequencies.
- Balance out the two hemispheres of the brain, again as measured by EEG tests.

- Work as an antidepressant since it inhibits the uptake of noradrenaline by PC12 nerve cells.
- And finally, there's cancer.

Cancer

That's right—as if all of the benefits we've listed so far were not enough. **The regular intake of Scalar Enhanced™ products may very well play a significant role in preventing and/or reversing cancer.**

Cancer cells are, almost without exception, low-voltage cells. As I mentioned earlier, the optimum cell voltage for most cells in the body is in the 70–90 millivolt range. Cancer cells are almost exclusively in the 15–20 millivolt range.

There have been many theories proposed as to why this is true. The most likely one is that as cell voltage starts to drop into the range where the very survival of the cell may be called into question, the cell begins to proliferate uncontrollably in an attempt to guarantee its "survival."

If you raise cell voltage (which is exactly what can happen when you consume Scalar Enhanced™ products), the cell no longer needs to proliferate wildly. In effect, it can become "normal" again. The implications for this in treating cancer could be profound.

Conclusion

How long will products hold their charge?

- The higher the quality of the product to start with, the longer it will hold a charge. High-quality "alive" organic type products actually will often display a stronger charge after 6 months then when first charged.

Are charged products safe?

- Absolutely. Again, there is nothing unnatural about scalar energy. It has been around since the creation of the universe. It's all a question of embedding healing/energizing frequencies as opposed to harmful frequencies.

Which frequencies do we embed?

- Without giving away proprietary information, there are two key frequencies focused on. First, is the Schuman Resonance. This is in the 7.8-8.0 HZ range. It is the frequency the earth emits when there is nothing around—nothing manmade and no plant or animal life around. It is the innate frequency of the earth. The other frequency is closer to 12 HZ. This is the frequency that you will record in a rainforest—again with nothing manmade around. These are the core scalar frequencies that accomplish everything we've talked about in this chapter.

What will I notice by using Scalar Enhanced™ products?

- In addition to every other benefit that I've outlined so far, you will find that scalar enhanced products will be absorbed faster, work faster, and produce stronger results.

What does this all mean?

- Scalar Enhanced™ products enter your body fast and work better than comparable nonenhanced products.
- Scalar Enhanced™ products charge every single cell of your body with health promoting scalar waves.
- The more Scalar Enhanced™ products you use and the more often you use them, the more profound the effect. The effect is cumulative.
- Someday, every nutritional company will scalar-enhance their products or they will not be able to stay in business. Scalar Enhanced™ products are simply that superior.

What will I notice by using Cedar Balsamea™ products?

- In addition to every other benefit that [illegible] you will find that [illegible] products [illegible] produc[illegible] [illegible]

What does this allow?

- [illegible] products [illegible] and [illegible]
- [illegible] products [illegible]
- [illegible]
- [illegible]

CHAPTER 18

LET'S TALK ABOUT CANCER

I'm not going to prescribe or play doctor in this chapter, merely explore the nature of the disease on a theoretical basis. Nevertheless, I think you will find that the mere act of exploration opens up a whole range of possible treatment options—once you understand the true nature of the disease.

First, let's talk about the state of cancer in the United States today.

If you believe what you read in the press, cancer treatment is making great strides.

- Diagnosis and treatment are better than ever.
- More people are being saved than ever before.
- People are living longer after diagnosis than ever before.
- Discovery of the cancer gene and the elusive "cure for cancer" are right around the corner.
- Things have never looked better for winning the war on cancer.

On the other hand, if you look just below the surface, you find an entirely different story.

- We spend $100,000,000,000.00 a year on cancer in the United States.
- In the Feb 9, 1994 issue of the *Journal of the American Medical Association,* the "War on Cancer" was declared a failure. "**In all age groups, cancer incidence is increasing . . . few new effective treatments have been devised for the most common cancers.**"
- The incidence of cancer is soaring—up between 800% to 1,700% in the last 100 years (depending on whose numbers you look at). According to the American Cancer Society, 1 in every 2.5 Americans (and moving rapidly to 1 in 2) will get some form of invasive cancer in their lives—and half of those who get it will die from it. (Now, it is true that the rates for some forms of cancer such as prostate cancer and colon cancer have dropped slightly in the last couple of years, but keep in mind that drop is only relative to the extremely high levels that were reached in the last 100 years and that the rates for other forms of cancer (such as lymph cancer) have soared—more than offsetting the small drops just mentioned.

- More people are dying than ever before from cancer. In the early 1900s, cancer was a rare occurrence in the American population. Today, it is the number 2 killer in the United States—trailing only heart disease.

So which story is true? They can't both be true. Can they?

Actually, they can—sort of. It all comes down to a statement attributed to Benjamin Disraeli, one of England's great Prime Ministers. According to Disraeli, "There are three kinds of lies in the world: lies, damn lies, and statistics." And that's exactly what we have here: statistical lies.

Just do a little logical thinking, and the truth begins to shine forth. So let's take these claims one at a time and see what the truth is behind them.

More People Are Surviving Cancer Than Ever Before

If mortality rates are virtually unchanged (as stated in the *Journal of the American Medical Association*), but 800 to 1,700 percent more people are getting cancer than ever before, then 8–17 times as many people will be saved—would they not? Thus the remarkable claims you see in the press.

On the other hand, what you don't hear as often is that 8–17 times as many people are also dying—whoops! Thus the rise of cancer to its position as the number 2 killer in the United States.[1]

So which is the most important statistic? Quite simply, none of them. It's the fact that survival rates are virtually unchanged. What that means is that modern medicine isn't really making much of a difference.[2]

People Are Living Longer with Cancer Than Ever Before

If better testing is diagnosing cancer earlier than ever before, then, by definition, people would be living longer than ever before after diagnosis, even with no real change in the effectiveness in treatment or the actual survival rate—would they not? Bottom line is that people are not really living longer. They're just being given a longer death sentence. Now it is true that the statistics claim to have accounted for this quirk. They haven't really. For one thing, they don't account for the number of people who die from the side effects of treatment.

---

[1]It's also worth keeping in mind that the population of the United States has increased 360% in the last hundred years (75,000,000 to 270,000,000). That means you can multiply both the survival and mortality rates by 3.6. In other words, the 8–17 times becomes 29–61 times. And that's how cancer has risen from virtual obscurity to become the number two killer in the USA, claiming several hundred thousand people a year.

[2]Mortality rates are actually worse than they first appear. Consider the fact that when a cancer patient undergoes chemo, and then succumbs to pneumonia because their immune system has collapsed from the chemo, that is recorded as death by pneumonia—not cancer. Now add in all of the people who have died from the side effects of chemo and radiation, and you find that mortality rates are not just unchanged but have probably gone backwards.

How Can This Be?

Are we being scammed and lied to? Are cures being deliberately suppressed, as some people believe?

Although many in the alternative health community believe otherwise, I think the answer to both questions is no. There is no scam, no deliberate suppression.

On the other hand, with $100,000,000,000.00 dollars being spent every year on cancer in the United States, cancer has become, quite simply, a major industry. And therein lies the problem. You now have vested interests competing for a piece of this monstrous pie. This leads to a series of major problems.

- No one has an interest in preventing cancer, since that doesn't produce any money. All interest is in finding "a cure for cancer." This is where the fame is. This is where career advancement is. And yes, this is where the money is.
- Any cure found must be proprietary—otherwise no money can be made.[1]
- Any cure must come from within the medical community—to justify all of the money being raised and spent—and, in fact, to justify the doctor's very existence as a doctor.[2]

That means that

- Even though it's relatively easy to reduce the incidence of cancer by close to 90% (back to the levels experienced 100 years ago), no one in the medical community will tell how. (Just remove the toxins from your body—toxins that didn't even exist 100 years ago but are now present in our bodies in substantial amounts, and start regenerating your body with the essential nutrients that have been removed from the mass produced, processed foods that make up the bulk of today's diet).
- Even though there are natural treatments that are at least as effective as chemo and radiation and surgery (not hard to do, since the medical modalities are so ineffective and have such deleterious side effects), no one in the medical community will tell you about them.

---

[1]And this is another area in which the deck is rigged against alternative treatments. Since it now takes several hundred million dollars to approve a new drug or treatment in the United States, any program that is not proprietary can never be approved, because no one can afford to take it through the testing process if they don't own the rights to it. When you hear drug companies complain about the high cost of drug approval, don't believe it. They love it. That's what keeps small players from disrupting their multi-billion dollar profit factory.

[2]Actually, this is probably the biggest single factor. In the end, ego is more important than money.

- Even though the concept of a "cure for cancer" is basically bogus (more on that later), you will still be asked to raise and contribute billions of dollars to search for it.[1]

So Let's Talk About the Nature of the Disease.

Does anyone really believe that **cancer somehow magically appears in isolated spots in your body for no particular reason? And that removing or destroying that cancer in that one isolated spot means that you're cured?**

Does the above statement sound silly, or even absurd, to you? If it does, you've got a problem. You see, virtually all modern cancer research and treatments are based on that premise.

- Surgically remove the cancer.
- Burn it out with focused beams of radiation.
- Poison it with chemo.
- Or all of the above.

If we want to end the cancer scourge, we need to look elsewhere for answers. And probably the best place to start is with a discussion of what cancer actually is.

What Is Cancer

Cancer is fundamentally a disease of the immune system. What do I mean by that? Quite simply, in your body, as part of the normal metabolic process, you produce anywhere from a few hundred to as many as 10,000 cancerous cells each and every day of your life.

So why doesn't everybody get cancer? Because your immune system has the ability to recognize each and every one of those aberrant cells and remove them from your body. That's what a healthy immune system does.

Then why do some people get cancer? Because one of three things happens (and more often than not all three together):

1. You expose yourself to toxins and outside influences (such as heavy metals, radiation, rancid fats, viruses, bacteria, parasites, etc.) that dramatically increase the number of cancerous cells your body produces so that not even a healthy immune system can handle the load.

---

[1] I know a woman who had breast cancer and had run through all the usual medical treatments to no avail. She was dying, and in fact, had been sent home to die by her doctors. As a last resort she went on the Baseline of Health program and experienced a total recovery. To celebrate her recovery, she now runs regularly in "Breast Cancer" races to raise money for research—and she's absolutely oblivious to the contradiction. God bless her!

2. You compromise your immune system to the point that it can no longer handle all of the cancerous cells your body produces—thus allowing some of them to take root and establish themselves.

3. Circulation (in the broadest sense) is impeded—thus leading to both 1 and 2 above.

Let's explore these three points in a little more detail.

1. Exposure to Toxins and Other Outside Influences

Some factors are known beyond a shadow of doubt; others are more hypothetical (but with strong circumstantial support).

- Exposure to radiation is an absolute known cause of cancer.
- Exposure to radon gas seeping up from the ground and into our houses is also a known cause.[1]
- Living in cities with polluted air like Los Angeles and Houston dramatically increase your chances of getting cancer. In fact, if you live in the Los Angeles basin, your chances of getting lung cancer are 426 times greater than if you live in an area with clean air.[2]
- There is now strong circumstantial evidence that transient viruses and bacteria are a major factor in producing cancer.
- Then again, we know that prolonged exposure to cigarette smoke is a known carcinogen.
- Chlorine in our water is a known carcinogen.
- Excessive estrogen is the only known cause of uterine cancer and plays a major role in several other kinds of cancer including breast cancer and prostate cancer.
- Improper elimination and the improper balance of beneficial bacteria in the colon are known cancer causers. And colon cancer is now the leading cancer among men and women combined.
- Excessive build-up of free radicals is a factor. Related to this, of course, is the consumption of rancid fats and transfatty acids.
- There are over 2,000 known carcinogens in our water supply.

---

[1]Radon gas is the number 2 cause of lung cancer in the US. Second only to smoking cigarettes according to the EPA, Surgeon General, and The American Lung Association. Millions of homes and buildings contain high levels of radon gas. http://www.epa.gov/iaq/radon/

[2]Although California has made strides in reducing hazardous air pollution, a Congressional Report released on 3/1/99 found toxins at high enough levels that the risk of cancer was 426 times higher than health standards established by the 1990 federal Clean Air Act.

- Even something as simple as repeated acid reflux will eventually stress the lining of the esophagus enough that esophageal cancer results.
- etc.

Does it sound overwhelming? In a sense it is. However, it's only overwhelming if you're looking for a magic bullet cure. In fact, simple protocols such as the Baseline of Health will eliminate virtually all of these factors from your body. Then the whole concept of preventing and reversing cancer becomes much more understandable.

2. Compromised Immune System

And how do we compromise our immune systems? As it turns out, almost every which way you can imagine.

- How good can your immune system be (taking all the supplements in the world that you want) if your colon is packed with 20 lbs of old fecal matter? A substantial portion of your immune system then has to combat the effects of self-toxicity. Clean up your intestinal tract, and you free up your immune system.
- Beneficial bacteria manufacture potent immune boosters such as Transfer Factor and Lactoferrin right in your intestinal tract—if they're there. In other words, the proper balance of beneficial probiotics in your intestinal tract can substantially boost your immune system by increasing internal production of a number of powerful immune factors. Without those factors, your immune system is marginalized.
- Taking digestive enzymes between meals relieves stress on the immune system by helping to eliminate Circulating Immune Complexes from the body. Given today's enzymatically dead diet, this is essential to prevent a total breakdown of your immune system.
- Proper diet and nourishment boost your immune system. Each and every immune cell in your body is manufactured from the food you eat. A nutritionally deficient diet means functionally deficient immune cells. The bottom line is that you can't build the same immune cell out of pepperoni pizza, beer, and twinkies that you can out of whole living foods. Supplementation with the proper vitamin and mineral complexes will significantly enhance the production of your body's immune cells.
- Deficiencies of the key fatty acids is a sure invitation to cancer. In fact, some of the fatty acids actually work as immune system modulators that help to keep the immune system properly programmed so it doesn't attack itself.

- A full spectrum antioxidant boosts the immune system in multiple ways. Just one example is Curcumin. In *Immunological Investigations,* 1999, Vol 28, Issue 5–6, pp 291-303, there are published studies that prove that Curcumin can increase white blood cell count by some 50% in just 12 days—not to mention circulating antibodies by some 512 in the same time frame.
- Cleaning out the liver improves its ability to produce immune factors and remove bacteria from the blood. An impaired liver is like a death sentence to your immune system.
- Cleaning out the blood and balancing your blood's pH also helps to improve immune function. In fact, low pH in body tissue is almost a guarantee for the onset of cancer.
- Invading pathogens can eventually overwhelm the immune system, rendering it incapable of performing its normal protective functions.
- Your mental attitude matters. There is a strong statistical correlation between depression and cancer.
- Lack of exercise reduces immune function and causes the lymph to stagnate—further compromising the immune system.
- And keep in mind that the ingredients in a single can of soda can depress parts of your immune system by as much as 50% for as long as 6 hours or more. So what does that mean if you drink 4–5 cans of soda a day—or more?

Again, what at first appears to be overwhelming becomes quite manageable when we view it as part of the whole.

3. Circulation

By circulation here, I'm using it in the broadest sense, as it applies to all of the body's circulatory systems: Blood, Lymph, and Energy.

Blood

If there is any restriction of blood circulation (caused by anything from narrowing of the arteries to tension in the surrounding muscle tissue) several problems arise.

- Sufficient oxygen can no longer reach key areas of the body. Oxygen is a cancer destroyer.
- Sufficient nutrients can no longer reach that area of the body, thus starving it, weakening it, and making it vulnerable to mutation.
- The waste material produced by the cells can no longer be efficiently removed. The build-up of toxic waste in the cells eventually leads to cancer.

Lymph

- Your lymph is your body's sewer system, removing dead cells, waste, toxic matter, heavy metals, bacteria, etc. from body tissue. Unfortunately, the lymph system has no pump of its own. If for any reason your lymph is stagnant, you end up poisoning yourself. Cancer is a likely outcome.

Energy

- Fundamentally, our bodies are pure energy systems. As you look more and more closely at the subatomic structure of all matter, the physical world begins to disappear. All that's left is a series of force fields and probabilities that create the illusion of matter as we know it. Certainly, we have to deal with this illusion (the physical world) as we see it, but we also have to deal with the consequences of the world of energy that remains unseen—but is nevertheless the true reality behind all physical matter. The bottom line is that a major factor in the onset of cancer is when these energies in our body become unbalanced or diminished in any way.
- And, as we learned in the last chapter, cancer cells are almost exclusively low-energy cells.

So Where Does That Leave Us?

Once we understand what cancer actually is, it's easy to understand:

- Why medical treatments for cancer have had such dismal results.
- Why most of the current research is a waste of time and money.
- And most important of all, what you can do to prevent and in many cases even reverse cancer.

So let's take on these points one at a time.

1. Why medical treatments for cancer have had such dismal results

This is real obvious. Medical treatments are based entirely on eliminating the symptoms (or manifestation) of the cancer in your body. They do nothing to eliminate the causes of cancer—to remove those things that stimulate it's growth in the body.

Think about this for a moment. Does surgery or radiation treatment or chemotherapy do one single thing for any of the causes that we have discussed in the previous sections? And the answer, of course, is zero, zilch, nada, nothing. All they do is attempt to remove the symptom (the physical manifestation of the cancer) that results from these causes. Is it any wonder they have had such a poor track record? And on top of everything else, now that we know the causes of cancer, we can see that radiation and chemo actually significantly compound the problem.

- Exposure to radiation is a known carcinogen. Every treatment increases the likelihood of future cancer.
- Chemo drugs are some of the most power carcinogens known. Think about this for a moment. The prime cancer treatment we use today actually fills your body with some of the most powerful **cancer-causing** drugs known. Whoa! Who came up with this treatment? The absurdity of it is mind boggling. Even if you temporarily destroy the current cancer in your body by poisoning it with these drugs, haven't you significantly increased your chances of getting cancer down the road?
- But it gets even worse. Medical treatments do nothing to improve immune function in the body. In fact, chemo and radiation quite literally destroy immune function in your body.[1] This is the single most absurd aspect of the modern medical approach to dealing with cancer—destroy the very system in your body that can actually eliminate and prevent the recurrence of that cancer, and then do nothing to repair that damage. At the very least, this is highly irresponsible.[2]
- And maybe, most damning of all, these treatments are deadly in and of themselves. Chemotherapy drugs are incredibly toxic. The fundamental premise behind their use is actually frightening. "We're going to give you some of the most powerful poisons we know in all creation. Why? Well, we hope your cancer will pull the poison in faster than the rest of your body—and therefore die before you do. Of course, if we're wrong, you'll die from the treatment and not your cancer. And at the very least, since it is so poisonous, you're going to feel really really ill—much worse than you've ever felt in your life. Your hair will fall out. You'll vomit repeatedly. You'll feel as though your very life is being drained from your body (which is actually what's happening). But, of course, it's worth it if it works. **And it is your only option.**" I don't know how many times I've seen people die from the chemotherapy and not the cancer. But two things, in particular, really gall me.
- First, I know of numerous cases where people have gone through chemo, and despite all the suffering it didn't work.[3] Unfortunately, the patients were so debilitated by the treatment, that another round of chemo was not an option.

---

[1]I have seen numerous examples of people who have chosen to use immune boosting formulas, such as Immunity Plus, while undergoing chemo and have actually seen their immune function not only **not** drop, but in fact, increase—even double—during the course of that chemo treatment.

[2]After we saw what Immunity Plus could do in concert with chemotherapy, I wrote to 6 major hospitals in the United States with complementary health programs and offered to fund a study that proved the benefits of immune system enhancement during chemo. Not one hospital responded. I wrote to each a second time. Again nothing. With the third letter, I finally got a response. Finally, one of the hospitals wrote back and told me to never write them again!

[3]In fact, the benefits of chemo vary widely from cancer to cancer—sometimes improving "short-term" survivability by as much as 50%; but also, in many cases, by 1% or less.

They were then "sent home" by their doctor to die. At that point, with no other options left to them, they tracked down one of the "miracle doctors." Amazingly, they began to feel better almost from day one. After a few weeks, they felt so much better that they went back to their original oncologist for a check-up. An exam showed no sign of cancer (or the cancer was dramatically reduced). The oncologist then proceeded to tell the patient that their alternative program had nothing to do with their recovery (bad enough in and of itself), but then went on to convince the patient to come back for another round of chemo to "make sure the cancer doesn't come back." And then the patient died of a heart attack as a side effect of that "insurance" chemo.

- Another variation of this which I have seen repeatedly is the patient who uses immune boosting formulas (such as Immunity Plus and liquid minerals) while undergoing chemotherapy. The results are far beyond what the doctor expects. The patient, in fact, tests cancer-free half way through the chemotherapy program. Nevertheless, the doctor insists on the last two or three rounds of chemo. And the patient dies as a result of the chemo in those final rounds.

2. Why most of the current research is a waste of time and money

This is magic bullet nonsense. Take the search for the cancer gene. Are there genes that give one a predisposition to getting cancer? Absolutely. This is exactly what the Baseline of Health talks about when it refers to your Personal Health Line at the time of birth. But looking for a cancer cure by finding the cancer gene will do nothing to eliminate all of the other factors that we know are responsible for cancer. And, in fact, we already know how small a role the "cancer gene" plays in the onset of cancer. There has been an 8–17-fold increase in the incidence of cancer in the last hundred years. Not even one-millionth of 1% of that increase can be related to genes. Genes evolve over hundreds of thousands (if not millions) of years. That means that the so-called cancer gene has had no impact on the huge increase we've seen since 1900. And that means that virtually 90% of all the cancer that we see today cannot possibly have anything to do with genes. And of that 10% that's left, only a certain percentage of that relates to the unknown cancer gene. That means, quite simply, that at best, genes were responsible for only a small percentage of the minimal cancer rates we had in the early 1900s, and that finding the "cancer gene" will affect only that tiny percentage of cancer. Bottom line: look not for a cure in the cancer gene.

3. What you can do: the alternatives

According to the medical establishment, there are no effective alternative treatments for cancer. Your only options are chemo, radiation, and surgery. In fact, in half the states in this country, it is illegal for even a medical doctor to prescribe anything other than chemo, radiation, or surgery as a treatment for cancer. The sad thing is that it absolutely is not true. There are effective alternatives.

But wait a second. Don't they test promising alternative therapies, and in each and every case find them invalid? And the answer is: yes, they test them, but skew the tests so that alternative therapies cannot pass. This is done in two ways.

The Whole Is Greater than the Sum of Its Parts

First, in almost all cases, alternative therapies are administered as **part** of a comprehensive program. Now that we've discussed the nature of the disease, it's easy to see why a comprehensive program is the only thing that makes sense. Nevertheless, when the medical community decides to test the validity of a particular treatment, they insist on separating out the pieces from the whole and testing them in isolation.

This would be akin to deciding to test a prospective football quarterback. The "alternative approach" would be to put him on the field with an entire team and see how he plays. The "medical approach" would be different. How can we really tell if he's any good if there are other players on the field? Great receivers could catch lousy passes and we'd never know. A great offensive line could make him look good by blocking so well that he had all the time in the world to find his receivers. No! The only way to truly tell if he's any good is to put him on the field alone against the entire all-pro defensive team. And, of course, the moment the ball is hiked, he's swarmed under and killed.

But then how do drugs pass this kind of testing? Quite simply, drugs are "magic bullets." In effect, they put him out on the field alone, but armed with an AK-47 assault rife. Of course, as soon as the ball is hiked, he shoots the entire defensive team and walks across the goal. Unfortunately, although he scores, there are side effects. The other team is dead, and the game is over—but he did score.

Look, just like football is a team game—with the team only as strong as it's weakest component—so too is alternative therapy for cancer a "team" program. On occasion, you may get good results using just one component or another, but overall you will get the best results when you run the program as a whole. To isolate components of a program from the whole is to treat them as drugs. That's not what they are, and they will fail that test by definition.

Additive vs Subtractive

In addition, medical treatments and alternative therapies are different in an even more fundamental way. Drugs are subtractive, whereas alternative therapies are additive.

- **Medical treatments such as chemo and radiation.**
  - As we've already discussed, medical treatments are subtractive in the very way they're evaluated. You subtract out every possible variable until you're left with the one active component.

  - Traditional medical treatments are an all or nothing proposition. If you use chemo, you wipe out your immune system, which pretty much ends the possibility of using your immune system to overcome the cancer. That means medical treatments have to work consistently in a high enough percentage of cases, or they are dismissed as invalid.[1] That makes sense when testing subtractive therapies like drugs, but makes no sense for testing alternative therapies. Nevertheless, that is the criterion used to evaluate alternative therapies.

- **Alternative therapies.**
  - Alternative therapies are not subtractive. They are "additive." Again, an alternative treatment that would be dismissed as ineffective because testing showed it to be only 10% effective in isolation, might nevertheless be an invaluable part of a comprehensive program that contained seven 10% components—giving you a 70% chance of overcoming your cancer. But the medical establishment deliberately chooses not to test alternative therapies in this way—thus condemning all seven components with the "quackery" label. So the only way you hear about effective alternatives is by word of mouth or anecdotal evidence. Fortunately, the effectiveness of some of these programs is so strong, that it is impossible to suppress their success. And that is why more and more people are turning away from the failing programs of the medical community and turning to effective alternatives.

Cost

And lest I forget, one of the biggest arguments against alternative therapies is that they are a waste of money. Please! We spend $100,000,000,000.00 a year on a medical war on cancer that has been declared a failure by its very generals. Spending $100 a month on supplements or even $2,000 for a Rife machine or an Ozone generator is a drop in the bucket compared to that obscenity. How unbelievably hypocritical to claim that they are trashing alternative therapies to protect your pocketbook!

General Recommendations

Preventing vs Reversing

It is much easier to prevent cancer than to reverse it. The reason is very simple. Isolated cancer cells are not very strong and have no built-in support mechanisms; however, once they take root and begin to multiply, they build awesome

[1]And even here, the medical establishment does not play with a full deck. Doctors routinely prescribe chemotherapy for advanced lung cancer cases where the success rate is less than 1%. Any alternative therapy with a 1% success rate would be laughed into oblivion by the establishment.

support systems, and acquire a life of their own. In the case of tumors, for example, this includes the development of fully functional, complex vascular systems capable of providing tremendous amounts of nutrition and sustenance—unfortunately at the expense of your body's vital organs. Also, once they take root, cancer cells are able to manifest their most important attribute—immortality. Unlike normal cells in your body, which have a limited life span (one of the main reasons we age and die), cancer cells, in general, do not age and die. Functionally, they can live forever. This gives them a major competitive advantage over healthy cells in your body.

The bottom line is that, yes, your body is capable of reversing an established cancer. Doctors see it all the time. They call it "spontaneous remission." But it is far easier to prevent cancer than it is to reverse it.

So what do you do to prevent or reverse cancer?

This is the big question, isn't it? Unfortunately, I cannot prescribe or recommend any particular treatments in this book. That would be against the law. However, it is not inappropriate to give you some guidelines.

Chemo, Radiation, and Surgery

First, surgery might play a role if a tumor were so large, for example, that it was impinging on another organ, thereby threatening near term death. In that case, surgery might make sense to give you the time to pursue alternatives.

On the other hand, I would be very leery of any chemo or radiation treatments. I would need to see very convincing (and I mean convincing) statistical evidence that those particular treatments were indeed effective for my particular type of cancer before I would even give them a passing look. Remember, chemo and radiation are "subtractive" treatments.[1]

The Alternatives

It's now time to take a look at the "additive" therapies—the therapies that remove the toxins from your body and build your body's natural defenses against cancer. They are additive in the sense that they can all build off each other. This is a very important concept so let me cover it once again. With chemo for example, if it gives you a 1% chance of success (as with most cases of advanced lung cancer), that's it. Since you've subtracted out all other options, those are your odds: 1 in 100. On the other hand, make use of an additive alternative treatment that has a 10% chance of helping you, and there's nothing stopping you from adding another treatment that also has a 10% success rate. Now you've got a 20% chance of success. And therein lies the secret to success.

---

[1]If you opt for chemo or radiation, it is absolutely imperative that you do something to repair your immune system concurrent with your treatment. Check with your doctor about using immune enhancers concurrently with your "therapy." They have consistently produced spectacular results in similar circumstances.

Do everything. Do it all at once. Do it intensively. And repeat it. And once you have the cancer on the run, keep doing it until there is no sign of cancer for at least 6 months. By everything, what do I mean?

- The Baseline of Health[1] program is specifically designed to clean out and nourish virtually every major system in your body. **It is by no means a cancer treatment. It is merely a system for optimizing the health of all the major systems in your body.** And it is for that reason that it serves as the core of any program you use to deal with catastrophic illness. It can play a significant role both in removing the toxins from your body that promote the growth of aberrant cells and in rebuilding and optimizing your immune system. Make sure you do every piece of the program—not just the convenient parts.[2] The liver cleanse and detox is crucial (particularly since it destroys parasites in the liver).[3] And don't forget things like taking the flaxseed, juice fasting, the mental exercises, and physical exercise. These are all key elements of the program.
- **Specific anti-cancer protocols to check out in the library or on the web**
  - Check out the Budwig diet.
  - Specialized antioxidants like curcumin, green tea, selenium, red raspberry ellagitannins, and L-carnosine should be explored.
  - Acemannan concentrates from aloe help build the immune system.
  - Ellagitannin extracts from red raspberries are proven powerful anticarcinogens.
  - Check out using high doses (12 tablespoons a day) of stabilized rice bran.
  - Check out Ukrain. This is expensive, but the results have been dramatic.
  - Check out Carnivora. This is much less expensive, but the first dose requires the administration of an injection. After that, all doses are oral.
  - Ozone Therapy. This therapy has been shown to be effective in burning cancers out of the body. It's administered using rectal insufflation. Unfortunately, the machines are not inexpensive—costing about $2,200.
  - Rife Technology. There are several machines that have expanded upon the work that Royal Rife initiated. The basic premise of his work is that cancers can be eliminated by frequencies tuned to the individual electromagnetic signature of that particular disease. The medical establishment and self-appointed quack busters really dislike these machines which cost close

---

[1]Following the Baseline of Health program is the best single method available for preventing cancer from taking root in your body. It also offers the best base from which to launch any program intended to reverse cancer once it has, in fact, taken root.

[2]When using the Baseline of Health as part of a program for reversing cancer, you need to do it completely (no exceptions), intensively and repeatedly.

[3]You should also eliminate all forms of propyl alcohol (internal and external) from your life since there are indications these may play a role in promoting the growth of parasites in the body.

to $2,000. Nevertheless, they work. Not as consistently as some proponents would have you believe (because it only addresses microbe induced cancers), but it does work and can be a powerful addition to any cancer therapy. www.biosolutions.cc.

- Track down a scalar energy charging chamber, or consume large amounts of scalar enhanced products to help raise cellular energy levels.

Is this a Cure for Cancer?

Let's be clear right off: anyone who says they have a cure for cancer is misinformed. I make this statement, not just to make the FDA happy, but because it is a simple impossibility—even within the medical community. When I see ads for hospital-based cancer programs where patients talk about being "cancer free" for 5 years or 7 years or whatever, I gag. The simple truth is that no one is cancer free—ever!

First of all, not everyone gets well—no matter what program they use. That's the nature of life. Sometimes it's simply because there are so many variables. For example, if your house is concentrating radon gas seeping up from the ground below, and you never checked for it and didn't know; why then, you could be doing any program in the world (from chemo to carnivora) and your odds of overcoming lung cancer would be significantly lessened. Then again, if you live in the middle of farm country and are continually exposed to pesticides, that too lessens your odds, no matter what you do. Or what if you had lived near Love Canal and were exposed to dioxin, or were one or Erin Brockovich's client's unknowingly exposed to Chromium 6 in your water, you were in trouble no matter what health program you went on. Sometimes you just don't know. **But even in those cases, your odds are still significantly better on a program designed to detoxify (remove those very toxins) from your body than on a program that adds more toxins to it.**

Also, it's important to remember that every single day of your life your body produces anywhere from a few hundred to as many as 10,000 cancerous cells as part of its normal metabolic processes. That means no one, by definition, can be cancer free, ever. The only question is: can your body deal with those cells and prevent them from taking root and multiplying? That's it, pure and simple.

Any program that reinforces your body in that agenda is good and will improve your odds **dramatically.** Any program that undermines it is "questionable." And that, dear readers, is why chemotherapy and radiation (at least in their current forms) will someday be considered a barbaric remnant of our medical past, like doctors not washing their hands before surgery and using mercury to treat syphilis.

CHAPTER 19

SPECIFIC RECOMMENDATIONS ON WHAT TO DO TO BUILD YOUR BASELINE OF HEALTH, DAY BY DAY

The secret to health, the secret to all of the success that the great miracle doctors share, is that they look to raise every inch of a person's Personal Health Line. If you do that, if you raise the entire line, the odds of good health (even of recovery from terminal disease) are remarkably favorable. If you want great health, if you want relief from illness that has not responded to traditional medicine, try using this program in cooperation with your physician. The results may very well astound you—and your doctor.

SUPPLEMENTS

Daily For Everyone

- The bedrock of your supplement program is a broad-based supplement. I recommend a biodynamically grown, living-food, multi-vitamin/mineral complex.
- One and a half tablespoons of golden flaxseed ground and mixed with juice twice a day—before breakfast and supper.
- A liquid trace mineral supplement.
- A good probiotic.
- Enzymes with every meal.
- A full-spectrum antioxidant.
- Immune booster and pathogen destroyer.
- Drink a minimum of 64 ounces of pure, pH optimized water a day.

Daily For Those Over 30

- Progesterone cream for both men and women.
- Testosterone balancing formula for both men and women.

Periodic

- 2–4 times a year: colon cleanse and detoxification program.
- 2–4 times a year: blood/liver detox.

If seriously ill, the detox programs above are to be done immediately—back to back. Then, take one week off and repeat, and repeat again as long as necessary.

- Four times a year: fast on fresh juices (absolutely not bottled or canned) for 3–7 days. If you prefer, you can combine the quarterly juice fasts with the colon and blood/liver detox programs.

Again, if seriously ill, start a juice fast immediately. Drink up to a gallon of fresh juice a day—an 8 ounce glass every hour you're awake.

Optional

- If needed, take a colon activator daily to avoid retaining fecal matter. Also, the worse you eat and/or the more contact you have with toxins, the more often you need to cleanse and detox.

Lifestyle Changes

Daily Exercise

Even if you are ill (especially if you are ill), you must exercise. If all you can do is hobble around the bed with a walker, do it. Do one lap around the bed the first day, and two the next.

Relaxation

- Meditate daily—morning and evening. At the end of each session, practice a healing visualization and affirmation.

Diet

- You know what to do. If you can't be perfect in your dietary habits, at least be better than you are now.
- If you have a really bad day (filled with chili dogs, beer, and ding dongs), do a one day juice fast the next day. Your body has a remarkable ability to repair itself—if you give it a chance.

If you are ill, you have no choice. You must totally clean up your act until you are well. No cooked foods. No processed foods. Lots of fruits and vegetables—especially juices.

Good Health and Long Life